No Longer Immune: A Counselor's Guide to AIDS

WITHDRAWN

Craig D. Kain, Ph.D.

Foreword by Bernard Siegel, M.D.

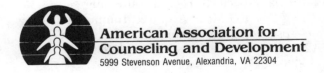
American Association for
Counseling and Development
5999 Stevenson Avenue, Alexandria, VA 22304

American Association for Counseling and Development
5999 Stevenson Avenue
Alexandria, VA. 22304

Library of Congress Card Number 89-6518

Printed in the United States of America
(Third Printing)
Cover design by Sarah Jane Valdez

Library of Congress Cataloging-in-Publication Data

No longer immune.

    Bibliography: p.
    1. AIDS (Disease)—Psychological Aspects. 2. AIDS
(Disease)—Social aspects. 3. Health counseling.
I. Kain, Craig D. [DNLM: 1. Acquired Immunodeficiency
Syndrome—psychology. 2. Counseling. WD 308 N739]
RC607.A26N6 1989   362.1′969792   89-6518
ISBN 1-55620-064-1

TABLE OF CONTENTS

SECTION FOUR
THE PROFESSIONAL CHALLENGES FOR
COUNSELORS

FOREWORD

AIDS. A scary word. It conjures up images of despair, loneliness and hopelessness. We are capable of erasing those images, and replacing them with caring, acceptance and understanding.

This book was written to help do just that. *No Longer Immune: A Counselor's Guide to AIDS* explores how to improve the physical, mental and spiritual well-being of HIV positive individuals. It emphasizes recognition and acceptance of the person behind the illness, and conveying that acceptance to the individual.

AIDS is not confined to one section of society: it is pervasive throughout. *No Longer Immune* addresses this fact and explores how society as a whole is becoming affected. Its broad coverage also examines the different segments of today's HIV positive population that have special needs, and addresses those needs. Women, children, families—no one will remain untouched by the epidemic.

Just as important as understanding the effects of AIDS on society today, is the history of the illness, and the outlook for the future. This publication provides background on AIDS, and then projects the implications it holds for the future. For only by facing the challenge head-on will we alter the destructive role this disease plays for the individual. The disease can be a gift for the individual and society for in the words of one individual, "AIDS was my cure, not my disease." AIDS healed his life and the by-product was a cure. Our goal must be to care for everyone, but we cannot cure everyone.

A book was sorely needed in order to educate and inform those in the helping professions on how to deal with AIDS. *No Longer Immune* is that book.

—Bernard Siegel, M.D.

INTRODUCTION

On a chilly night, in April of 1988, University of California at Los Angeles' Pauly Pavilion stood magestically. The pavilion, home to UCLA's title-winning basketball teams, was, on that night, hosting a different event. Around the outer perimeter of the upper row of bleachers hung, as always, large blue and gold banners, bold reminders of past championship seasons. On that night, new banners joined their ranks.

Spread out across the wooden floor and around the room itself were hundreds of new "banners" to be unveiled in the course of the evening. Each banner honored a player whose career had ended not with a win but rather with a loss. Throughout the night, these new banners, panels of a quilt that less than 6 months before had covered the mall from the Washington Monument to the Lincoln Memorial, were revealed, each bearing the name, artifacts, and memories of a person dead from AIDS.

Hundreds of men, women, and children were eulogized. Their names were sewn into the cloth, along with pictures, ribbons, and sequins. Hundreds of men, women, and children, witnesses to the Names Project AIDS Quilt's arrival in Los Angeles, gasped and cried as each name on each panel was read aloud.

In the course of the night, one man, an actor, rose to take his place in center court. He spoke eloquently, sharing his own battle against the toughest of all opponents, AIDS. He spoke of his hopes and dreams of beating the illness. He spoke of his despair at having watched so many of his friends and loved ones die while the government stood by not wanting to help. And, in the course of his speech, he uttered the message that would become the basis for this book. He stood there that night, looking out across the people in the stands, and said, "We all have AIDS." He reminded us that AIDS was not the problem of those who had died nor his problem, but our problem.

Acquired immune deficiency syndrome is everyone's crisis. Gone are the days of thinking of AIDS as a gay disease, a disease for drug users, a disease that no one we know will get. Gone are the days when only a handful of counselors would work with people with AIDS. The AIDS epidemic has changed, has grown, has mutated and exploded to the extent that today, counselors are no longer immune. We can no longer escape our responsibility to work with clients concerned or frightened or hurt or infected by AIDS. AIDS, a disease of the body's immune system, has affected the field of counseling in ways so crucial that we can no longer sit back as innocent bystanders. We must act. We are no longer immune.

Once we recognize and accept the premise that we are no longer immune, we are drawn to act, compelled to act. In their book, *How Can I Help?*, Paul Gorman and Ram Dass wrote that "'how can I help?' is a timeless inquiry of the heart." *No Longer Immune: A Counselor's Guide to AIDS* attempts to answer that question by looking at what we, as counselors, must do in the face of the worsening AIDS crisis.

Explicit in its title is the notion that this book is a guide. A guide can be many things. A guide can be a person who shows others the way. A guide can be one whose job involves pointing out sights on a journey. A guide can be a thing that marks a position. A guide can be an advisor, a person or thing that directs or influences one's behavior. *No Longer Immune: A Counselor's Guide to AIDS* is all of these. The 14 chapters that compose the book show counselors a way through the overwhelming complexity of the AIDS crisis. Some chapters point out sights, important issues for counselors to be aware of and, just like sights on other journeys or vacation trips, not all are beautiful. Some chapters mark a position, telling us where we are now in the scope of the crisis and where we will have to go in the future. Almost every chapter advises, directing counselors toward a way in which they can become more personally involved with AIDS work.

This book is a guide for those who "counsel." Throughout the book the term "counselor" or "counseling" is used, although not in an exclusive way. The authors of the book recognize that many people counsel, many people help others to recognize their full potential. Certainly, psychologists, counselors, and therapists counsel. So, too, do social workers. Physicians and nurses working with people with AIDS also find themselves in the role of counselor. Educators and clergy are counselors as well. The friends and family of a person with AIDS can at times be the best counselors he or she may ever have. This book is for all of them, for all counselors, whether they call themselves a counselor or just someone who cares and wants to help.

Compiling a guide to AIDS is not an easy job. The AIDS crisis is constantly changing. What was an established fact yesterday is a past theory today. The scope of the crisis is so broad that it is impossible to include everything in one book and still have the volume be readable (let alone something a reader could pick up without risking a hernia). Given that, this book presents the most comprehensive overview possible of the AIDS crisis today as we enter into the 1990s.

A number of considerations went into the design of this book. It was important that each author be an expert in his or her respected area of AIDS work. The contributors are leaders in their fields, writing, lecturing, and organizing at the forefront of the AIDS crisis. In keeping with the theme that no counselors remain immune, it was important that the contributors represent a broad cross section of geographical locations and work sites. The contributors live and work in places as metropolitan as San Francisco and as rural as Valdosta, Georgia. They work in hospitals and in private practice, in universities and in parishes.

No Longer Immune: A Counselor's Guide to AIDS is divided into 4 sections. The first section provides a foundation for the rest of the book. Chapter 1 on emergent trends surveys the sociological and psychological development of the AIDS crisis in the 1980s. It also sets the stage for the future developments of the crisis in the 1990s. Chapter 2, a companion chapter to the first, reviews psychosocial AIDS research. The two chapters together offer readers unfamiliar with AIDS an excellent place to start.

The second section is devoted to issues arising from working with specific populations. Although many issues cross sex, age, class, and cultural and sexual orientation distinctions, many do not. Chapter 3 takes a generalist's view of working with a person who is seropositive with respect to the AIDS virus. This chapter looks at both people who are symptomatic, showing signs of AIDS infections, and those who are asymptomatic. The next four chapters examine issues specific to particular populations. Chapter 4 looks at working with women. Chapter 5 considers how to approach adolescents with the realitites of the AIDS crisis. Chapter 6 presents the plight of the substance user. Chapter 7 examines how counselors can take a culturally sensitive approach to their AIDS counseling.

The book's last two sections examine special issues. The third section examines special issues for people with AIDS. The four chapters of this section cover psychoneurological issues (chapter 8), working with families (chapter 9), the role of the hospice (chapter 10), and spiritual issues (chapter 11).

The final section of the book is devoted to special issues for counselors. The three chapters of this section describe issues that directly affect the caregiver. Chapter 12 examines the counselor's role as educator. Chapter 13 clarifies the legal and ethical considerations that accompany AIDS work. The book's final chapter is a confronting and moving consideration of countertransference issues that arise when counselors work with people with AIDS.

Throughout the book, the authors stress that counselors should not operate in a vacuum. Counselors need not feel as though they are the only ones doing the difficult and demanding work of helping people with AIDS. The authors of this book, drawing from their own personal experience, repeatedly advocate networking. Counselors working with people with AIDS need to talk to and be supported by other counselors. "Resources for Counselors," at the end of this book, provides a state-by-state listing of some of the major community-based AIDS service providers. These organizations are the perfect place for counselors to form counselor support systems. They are also a great place to obtain current AIDS information. Counselors looking for referral agencies should find this list helpful. Perhaps most importantly, these organizations provide a setting for counselors who are willing to get involved and offer their services.

Each author expresses the hope that counselors will take a more active role in working toward the prevention of the misery and heartbreak that is the AIDS crisis. Participation on the part of the counseling profession is mandatory. We must combat our feelings of immunity to involvement. It is my hope that *No Longer Immune: A Counselor's Guide to AIDS* will serve as a true guide, a road map of sorts, leading readers to the path of compassion and action.

Much time and effort goes into putting together a book like this. I extend many people my heartfelt appreciation. A book is only as good as its contributors, and I was fortunate to have had the opportunity to work with knowledgeable and devoted people. My thanks go out to each author for his or her hard work, caring, and selflessness in agreeing to donate their proceeds from this book to the people who need it most, people with AIDS. I am, of course, indebted to the American Association for Counseling and Development for taking on the responsibility of publishing this book. I am also grateful to the people at AACD, particularly W. Mark Hamilton, Nancy Garfield, Lori Rogovin, and Rod Goodyear for their personal assistance. My thanks to Janine Bernard (Fairfield University), Fernando Guttierrez (The Growth Center, Santa Clara, CA), Barbara Kerr (University of Iowa), Ian Stulberg (Sherman Oaks Community Hospital), and Phyllis Gillman (private practice) who acted as reviewers for this book. Peter Lee of the National AIDS Network was a lifesaver in providing the material for the resources list. Melissa Johnson offered her critical comments throughout the project. Guy Lewis and Neil Fenn offered their support and caring during my darkest times. I am thankful to Neil Einbund, whom I consider not only a friend but a brother. My family, Bette, Richard, and Cindy constantly helped me to keep this project in perspective, reminding me not to take it seriously when I was overstressed and to take it seriously when I downplayed the importance of the work I was doing. Finally, I am indebted, beyond words, to the source of love and light in my life without whom this book would not exist.

—*Craig D. Kain*

Section One

OVERVIEW

Section Introduction

Before beginning or continuing on a journey, a person often finds it necessary to pause and take account of where he or she has arrived and where he or she intends to go. Counselors who have been deeply involved with AIDS work, and those who merely anticipate becoming involved, need to assess the current scope of the AIDS crisis. Thus, *No Longer Immune: A Counselor's Guide to AIDS* begins with an overview section that reviews the first years of the AIDS epidemic and anticipates the prominent issues that counselors will face in the coming years.

In the book's opening chapter, Kain reviews the significant medical, political, social, educational, and psychological events of the AIDS crisis. He relies on the concept of emergent trends to tie together the events of the first 10 years of the epidemic. Kain then turns to the decade of the 90s and suggests 10 areas of importance to counselors. These future trends set the tone for the rest of the book; many are examined in their own individual chapters in the book's other sections.

In chapter 2 Guydish and Ekstrand provide an in-depth review of psychosocial research on HIV spectrum disease. This chapter is clinically focused and surveys literature on HIV epidemiology, persons at risk for AIDS, asymptomatic seropositive persons, and people diagnosed with AIDS or ARC. The central theme of this chapter, as in many of the other chapters to follow, is prevention, which continues to be the greatest hope counselors have for slowing the continual spread of AIDS.

Both chapters describe AIDS work in its broadest scope. Together, these chapters emphasize the major thrust of *No Longer Immune: A Counselor's Guide to AIDS*: counselors must become involved.

Chapter 1

EMERGING TRENDS: AIDS TODAY AND IN THE FUTURE

Craig D. Kain

It is hard to believe that nearly 10 years have passed since the first immune-suppressed man asked for help. For tens of thousands of men, women, and children touched and torn by acquired immune deficiency syndrome (AIDS), the 80s was a decade where the passage of days, years, and lives was seen with crystalline clarity. There existed a heightened awareness of living on what Monette (1988) described as "borrowed time." Many things have changed in those 10 years; many things have not.

In its broadest sense, this chapter reviews the history of AIDS. To work effectively counselors must have a historical and societal context in which to place their clients and themselves. Examining the course of AIDS in the 80s reveals a number of trends. Five categories, though hardly distinct, emerge, offering a framework from which to examine these trends. The AIDS epidemic has affected science and medicine, politics, society, education, and counseling. Although these affected areas show considerable overlap, they will be discussed as separate entities in the course of this chapter.

Looking at the past is necessary, yet hardly sufficient. Counselors know that to get stuck in the past is to lose sight of the future; with AIDS the future is where hope lies. The second part of this chapter looks ahead, attempting to foreshadow crucial developments in the AIDS crisis and the impact they may have on counselors and other human development specialists.

Although examining the past and forecasting the future are the stated goals of this chapter, another subtler purpose

exists. In the 1990s many new therapists and counselors will
have to confront AIDS issues in their work. It will be important
for them to have a strong background and understanding of
what constitutes "the specter of AIDS" (Simon, 1988). Counselors who have had little experience with AIDS work will find
that this chapter provides them with an introduction and explanation of terms, concepts, and issues. Counselors familiar
with AIDS will find that this chapter offers them a concise
overview and a challenging preview of the future.

AIDS In the Eighties

An Emergent Trend in Science and Medicine:
The Language of AIDS

AIDS caught the medical profession off guard, coming at
a time when epidemiologists believed that infectious disease no
longer posed a threat to the developed world. Noninfectious
conditions such as cancer, heart disease, and degenerative diseases were thought to pose the remaining menace to the public
health (Gallo & Montagnier, 1988). AIDS changed these assumptions, creating a major medical catastrophe (Altman, 1986).
At the end of the 80s there was no cure, no antidote, and
no vaccine for AIDS. The decade's "major" advances, the discovery of the virus believed to cause AIDS and the use of AZT
and other experimental drugs to prolong the life of people with
AIDS, pale in comparison to the increased severity of the epidemic. Even Gallo and Montagnier, the investigators responsible for establishing the cause of AIDS, remarked that "in some
respects, the virus has outpaced science" (1988, p.41).
What, then, have medical and scientific researchers contributed to the fight against AIDS? Their largest contribution
lies in the lexicon of words and phrases that has emerged as a
way of describing, characterizing, and communicating AIDS.
Language, though often taken for granted, provides a tool for
conceptualizing the unknown. In this ability to construct the
world, language is most powerful. Words given to the epidemic
from the very start have helped to shape, sometimes in dele-
terious ways, the course of the crisis we call AIDS.
The language of AIDS began with a small, almost un-
noticeable report in the July 4, 1981, issue of the Center for

Disease Control's *Morbidity and Mortality Weekly Review*. The report outlined common symptoms of patients in New York City and California suffering from **Kaposi's sarcoma** and **pneumocystis pneumonia.** Until that time these terms were rarely used, referring to diseases that were seldom seen by doctors and certainly not in a fatal configuration. Kaposi's sarcoma, purplish lesions or patches appearing on the skin and affecting other organs like the lungs, heart and, most often, the lymph nodes, was known long before AIDS existed; it was an exceptional disease found in older subjects of Mediterranean descent and was usually "tranquil" (Leibowitch, 1985). Similarly, pneumocystis, a pneumonia caused by microorganisms, was, prior to AIDS, rarely seen (Osborn, 1987). The Center for Disease Control's (CDC) report marked Kaposi's sarcoma (**KS**) and pneumocystis (**PCP**) as entries into the language of AIDS.

As the number of cases of Kaposi's sarcoma and pneumocystis increased, a new term was added to the AIDS dictionary, with detrimental consequences. In the year following the first report by the CDC, the Center began referring to "homosexual or bisexual men" when speaking about the illnesses. It would have been far more appropriate for the CDC to speak of particular *behavior* as opposed to *identity*, and its failure to do so set the tone for the first name for what is currently known as AIDS: **GRID—gay-related immune deficiency.**

Although the term GRID was not specifically used by the CDC, it, or variations on the theme (i.e., "gay plague") soon came into common use. This emphasis on the gay aspects of the disease affected early research on AIDS; instead of focusing on a specific organism responsible for GRID, researchers looked for factors in the "gay life style" to explain what was going on (Altman, 1986). Even today, public perception of the disease and its sufferers continues to be affected by the term GRID's reference to sexual orientation.

The term GRID gave way to its logical heir, **AIDS**, **acquired immune deficiency syndrome**, a term used to describe a virtual smorgasbord of illnesses including KS and PCP as well as **toxoplasmosis**, **thrush**, and **cytomegalovirus**. The term AIDS quickly spawned a related term, **ARC—AIDS-related complex**. Doctors used this acronym to describe patients who demonstrated many debilitating symptoms like fever and sweats, general persistent fatigue, and persistent diarrhea and swollen glands, but failed to qualify for an AIDS diagnosis under the CDC's guidelines, which demanded the appearance of an **"opportun-istic disease."** This high-gloss term euphemistically referred to a host of disfiguring and destructive diseases that prey on weakened immune systems.

As medical research progressed, attention turned from genetic hypotheses for AIDS, linked to some innate homosexual predisposition, and from life-style hypotheses, linked to particular locations frequented only by gay men (Altman, 1986), to a viral cause for AIDS. This viral hypothesis, currently in popular acceptance, added three more terms to the dictionary of AIDS. Due to the particular political nature of the discovery of the AIDS virus, three separate names were used to designate what is and was the same virus. The American research team claimed the virus was **HTLV-III**, a distant relative of the HTLV (human T-lymphotropic virus), discovered by the National Institute of Health's Gallo. The French named their version of the virus **LAV** (lymphadenopathy associated virus), declaring their discovery a year before that of Gallo's was announced. Finally, an international commission changed the name to **HIV**, **human immunodeficiency virus**, eliminating the confusion caused by two names for the same entity (Gallo & Montagnier, 1988).

Although the research and consequent isolation of the HIV offered no immediate solutions to the crisis of AIDS, they did force new words into the vocabulary of the layperson. It was clear that the HIV virus was a **retrovirus**, a virus coded in the RNA of a cell as opposed to the DNA of a cell. The virus targeted the specialized **T-4 lymphocyte** cells, the cells responsible for the proper functioning of the body's immune system, and annihilated them.

Soon after the discovery of the AIDS agent, a laboratory test was developed to detect antibodies to HIV in the blood. This test, the **enzyme-linked immunosorbent assay (ELISA)** test, was created for the country's blood banks in an effort to keep the nation's blood supply free from AIDS. This, however, was not the only way the test came to be used. Individuals began relying on the test to assess their exposure to AIDS. Getting **"tested"** took on new meaning in the sociopolitical culture of the 80s. This popular use of the ELISA test resulted in new connotations for the terms **"seronegative"** and **"seropositive."** These terms, used to describe the lack of antibodies, or the presence of such antibodies, now implied life and impending death.

Although a positive result to the antibody test meant a person had been exposed to the virus, it did not mean a person had AIDS. Being **asymptomatic**, without overt warning signs, implied possible infectiousness, although at a rate thought to be less than that of symptomatic individuals (Heyward & Curran, 1988).

As the medical knowledge of AIDS increased, so too did the use of new terms describing the new situations that arose. Doctors as well as politicians, public health officials, counselors, reporters, and the public at large began to talk of **"risk groups," "the worried well,"** the **"exchange of bodily fluids,"** and **"safer sex."** AIDS patients were renamed **PWAs**, **people with AIDS**, in an effort to remove the notion of victimization.

To combat the ravaging illness that affected the men, women, and children with AIDS, medical researchers began pulling existing drugs off their shelves, trying anything reasonably likely to help those infected. Each drug added an additional entry into the growing AIDS dictionary. Although **AZT**, (**zidovudine**), the first effective anti-AIDS agent, brought hope that AIDS would not remain incurable forever (Gallo & Montagnier, 1988), its toxic side effects made it less than perfect, and certainly not the final answer (Yarchoan, Hiroaki, & Broder, 1988). By its direct antiviral action and by its partial restoration of immune functions, AZT may have a great effect if given early in the course of HIV infection, possibly preventing the progress of AIDS in some individuals (Yarchoan et al.). In addition to AZT, **CD4** seems to be a promising agent, serving as a viral receptor binding to the HIV, thus preventing it from infecting new cells (Gallo & Montagnier). **Aerosal pendamidine** and **dextran sulfate** also appear on the list of promising drugs. Additions to this list will be tempered by the fact that HIV appropriates the biosynthetic apparatus of the host cell. This means that drugs effective against the HIV tend to damage the host. Any vaccine must also take into consideration the HIV's capacity to integrate into the chromosomes of the host cell.

Implications for counseling. Counselors will need to keep familiar with current discoveries in the field of medicine and science. For many, this will be like learning a foreign language, with new diseases and new drugs added daily to their vocabulary. Clients with AIDS or at risk for AIDS are inundated with these terms and often use them as a way of describing their physical and *psychological* state. If counselors are to understand their clients, they must understand their clients' language.

An Emergent Trend in Politics: Resistance

Since first recognized, AIDS has been not solely a medical crisis but a political crisis as well. AIDS affects stigmatized segments of society, making the politicization of the syndrome more serious. Prejudice confounds and clouds politics, making the politicization more tragic. Emerging from the tangled web of political pomp and circumstance is the trend toward resistance.

Resistance takes on many shades and meanings. Resistance is an influence that hinders progress, as counselors working with highly resistant clients are aware. Another meaning of resistance refers to an organization or movement opposing the authorities. Both uses of the word fit the AIDS crisis. In the political arena, many people have hindered and opposed progress. In sharp contrast, the people most affected by AIDS have undertaken the formation of resistance movements, working for positive change.

AIDS is, in its purest sense, a bipartisan issue affecting Republican and Democrat alike, infecting liberals and conservatives without discrimination. However, to ignore the fact that the onset of AIDS occurred in the first year of the Reagan administration would be an oversight. The Reagan administration responded to the AIDS epidemic with great resistance, attesting to the notion that the politicization of AIDS reflects the circumstances of American politics in the 80s (Altman, 1986).

To look at AIDS and the government is to look at the availability of money for research, money for education, and money for prevention. Although the AIDS epidemic quickly fostered a volunteer response, particularly in gay communities hardest hit, which exemplified the kind of communal grass-roots organizing Reaganism extolled, the Reagan presidency was committed to trimming the financial fat off the country's budget, resulting in considerable cutbacks in funds available for both medical care and research (Altman, 1986).

In March of 1983, the Public Health Service issued the first risk-reduction guidelines in the federal government. "Sexual contact should be avoided with persons known or suspected to have AIDS" and "Members of high-risk groups should be aware that multiple sexual partners increase the probability of developing AIDS" represented the sum total of the U.S. government's attempt to prevent the spread of acquired immune deficiency syndrome almost 20 months after the original alert to AIDS (Shilts, 1988).

The outpouring of attention to the handful of heterosexual cases in early 1985 proved crucial in changing the lagging pace of the government's response to AIDS (Shilts, 1988). The widespread talk of heterosexual transmission of AIDS seized government officials, lending support to the notion that viewing AIDS as a "gay disease" was, until then, at least in part, responsible for the tepid response of the government.

Although funds became increasingly available as the number of heterosexual AIDS cases grew, the Reagan administration's resistance to a wholehearted commitment to prevent AIDS still showed. In 1985, Reagan asked the U.S. Surgeon General, C. Everett Koop, a recognized conservative, for a report on AIDS. Koop's report sat on the president's desk for 18 months before Reagan finally addressed it at the Third International AIDS Conference (Schram, 1988).

Later, in 1987, the president created his own commission on AIDS, which, after many politically motivated reorganizations, was finally chaired by Admiral James D. Watkins. The commission reported that "as long as discrimination occurs and no strong national policy with rapid and effective remedies against discrimination is established, individuals who are infected with HIV will be reluctant to come forward for testing, counseling and care" (Schram, 1988). The commission recommended that the president issue an executive order banning discrimination on the basis of considering HIV infection as a handicapping condition; the president responded by ordering yet another study, this one on discrimination (Schram).

The Congress too, became embroiled in political battles over AIDS. AIDS legislation, passed toward the end of Congress's 100th session, was the *first* comprehensive federal response to the AIDS epidemic since it was identified at the beginning of the 80s (Molotsky, 1988). The one billion dollar plan established prevention programs, developed care and treatment networks, and accelerated research efforts to find vaccines and cures. It did not, however, ensure confidentiality for patients whose tests showed they were carrying the disease, nor did it provide comprehensive education and mental health components. As it stood, the "AIDS Amendments Act of 1988" was, according to Lori Rogovin, a Washington lobbyist for the American Association for Counseling and Development, a "compromise" bill at best, sadly marking only a beginning step to the many issues surrounding the AIDS epidemic (personal communication, October 25, 1988).

Resistance could also be observed in the search for new biotechnology to combat AIDS in the 1980s. Like funding, new drugs and vaccines were political issues. In the United States, the release of new drugs into the common marketplace falls under the auspices of the Food and Drug Administration (FDA). Under FDA regulations, three phases of drug testing occur. Phase I trials, of short duration and involving a small number of patients, are designed to determine the safe dose range of a new drug and how the body deals with it. Phase II trials aim at determining whether a new drug has therapeutic efficacy and usually involve several hundred volunteers. Tests at this phase are controlled using a double blind regimen in which neither doctors nor patients know who receives the experimental drug or the control. Phase III trials typically include thousands of volunteers at multiple research centers and help to further define how and when a drug is optimally safe and effective (American Foundation for AIDS Research, 1988). Not until the end of 1988 did the FDA decide to revise new drug approval procedures in an attempt to make new treatments available more quickly to people with AIDS. Until the FDA revisions went into effect, the average time for the approval of drugs was 8 years (Leary, 1988). This stands in stark contrast to other countries, most notably France, home to the Pasteur Institute, one of the world's most important centers for treatment research. The French eagerly tested all sorts of drugs on AIDS patients, cognizant that the alternative to treatment was death (Shilts, 1988). Pasteur doctors considered Americans barbarous for not aggressively pursuing every possible means of treatment and considered double blind studies cruel and inhumane in that they precluded the patient who received a placebo from any chance of survival (Shilts).

Resistance to AIDS was not merely restricted to the legislative branches of government and its affiliated agencies. The press, watchguard of the government, was admittedly lax in its coverage of AIDS.

In the early days of the epidemic the media shied away from AIDS. In 1982 the *Morbidity and Mortality Weekly Report* announcement about KS received a one-day infusion of press attention and garnered obligatory stories in the *New York Times* and the *Los Angeles Times*, carefully crafted so as not to offend or cause panic (Shilts, 1988). By contrast, the discovery of cyanide in Tylenol capsules, which occurred at the same time, prompted the *New York Times* to write a story on the scare every day for the entire month of October and produce 23 more pieces in the 2 months following (Shilts). In *And the Band Played On*, Shilts wrote that in 1982 "one could have lived in New York, or in most of the United States for that matter, and not even have been aware from the daily newspapers that an epidemic was happening, even while government doctors themselves were predicting that the scourge would wipe out the lives of tens of thousands" (p. 191).

Political factors also influenced how reporters covered the AIDS crisis. Altman (1986) suggested that for the most part, the media avoided AIDS because they viewed it largely as a gay story. Once the illness appeared among infants and those who had received blood transfusions, attitudes changed dramatically. From early 1983 on, AIDS became a continuing preoccupation of the media. However, by that time the media had firmly established the homosexual character of the disease and the discovery of other affected groups changed this perception little (Altman, 1986).

Shilts (1988) pointed out that reporting on AIDS clearly followed a pattern; the stories were carefully written not to cause fear and always ended on a note of optimism. Virtually every news story stressed that AIDS was not casually infectious and that it posed no threat to the general public. Absent from early media coverage were clearly presented discussions of the specific sexual practices that spread AIDS, most notably anal intercourse.

While the federal government and media struggled to come to grips with the AIDS crisis, those closest to the illness formed politically oriented grass-roots movements. This active resistance movement was seen in candle-lit marches across the country, in demonstrations and rallies, in the thousands and thousands of handmade panels of the eulogistic "Names" quilt that filled the Washington mall in October 1987. Organizations like MAP, Mothers of AIDS Patients, called attention to the impact of AIDS on families during the 1988 presidential campaign while ACT-UP, the AIDS Coalition to Unleash Power, advocated civil disobedience as a way of channeling their growing anger over what they viewed as a maddeningly slow research effort.

Implications for counseling. Counselors need to be aware that their clients with AIDS or at risk for AIDS live in what has been a politically hostile environment. PWAs' lack of political power

is often internalized, resulting in feelings of helplessness, hopelessness, and despair. Counselors need to empower their clients,
combating resistance on the political and psychological fronts.
Counselors need to examine their role in the political apathy
toward AIDS and the impact their own political resistance may
have on the lives of their clients.

An Emergent Trend in Society: Dealing With the Disenfranchised

Society has often struggled with ways of dealing with the
disenfranchised, the segment of people who, for whatever reason, are discarded by the majority. AIDS confronted society
with an inordinate challenge—attending to stigmatized people
with life threatening illnesses. In the 1980s two major trends
in "coping" with the societal aspects of AIDS emerged, prejudice and caring.

The early days of the AIDS epidemic provided the raw
materials for the fear and prejudice that have become so deeply
ingrained in the crisis. Characterizing risk groups by the four
H's—homosexuals, heroin addicts, hemophiliacs, and Haitians—instead of by riskiness of behaviors, further stigmatized
already stigmatized groups.

Gay men suffered perhaps the most blatant forms of prejudice and hatred. Graffiti bearing messages like "AIDS—Americans' Ideal Death Sentence" became common (Altman, 1986).
Columns in newspapers bore headlines like "AIDS Disease: It's
Nature Striking Back," and argued that gays should be banned
from such activities as food handling and child care (Altman).
Stulberg and Smith (1988) reported that almost one fifth of the
gay men they sampled had experienced discrimination specifically as a result of AIDS. A survey done in October, 1988, by
the *New York Times* and *CBS News* reported that whereas most
respondents expressed sympathy toward people with AIDS in
general, they expressed little or no sympathy toward people
who get AIDS from homosexual activity (Kagay, 1988).

Prejudice against gays was not limited to the general pop-
ulace but occurred in the medical profession as well. An editorial by Dr. James Fletcher appeared in the *Southern Medical
Journal*, the official publication of the Southern Medical Association, claiming that "homosexuality is not 'alternative' behavior at all, but as the ancient wisdom of the Bible states, most

certainly pathologic" (in Altman, 1986). Baumgartner (1985) reported on health care professionals who, because of their discomfort in dealing with AIDS patients, enforce excessive infection control practices that leave their patients in isolation.

Haitians, too, suffered from incredible intolerance as a result of being included as a risk category. Whereas the media and researchers rushed to investigate every aspect of gay male life and how it had been affected by the epidemic, Haitians attracted far less attention (Altman, 1986). The classification of Haitians stirred controversy centering on whether it was correct to regard a nation as a whole as being at risk for AIDS. Dissenters claimed that a large percentage of Haitians were either homosexual or drug users and that the CDC ignored this due to a lack of interviewers skilled in Creole and aware of Haitian taboos (Altman). Although Haitians were eventually removed from the list of high-risk groups by the CDC, this extrication did little to alter the everyday discrimination AIDS presented for Haitians in North America (Altman).

Hemophiliacs risked exposure to the HIV virus through their use of Factor VIII, a product used to help clotting that is made from the plasma of large numbers of donors. Hemophiliacs became more inclined to hide their illness after the onset of the AIDS crisis, fearing exposure to the same sorts of prejudice other risk groups experienced (Altman, 1986).

Prejudice also emerged in the form of racism. Both within and outside the gay community, AIDS has been seen as largely a White disease resulting in a lack of comprehensive education and prevention programs as well as medical, psychological, and other support services directed specifically at people of color. This occurred despite the high incidence of AIDS among Black and Hispanic men (Altman, 1986).

Not all of society responded to AIDS with fear, loathing, and hatred. One of the most remarkable byproducts of the HIV epidemic was the development of community-based organizations dedicated to serving the needs of people with AIDS (Fineberg, 1988). These organizations, many of them nonprofit and locally organized, provided thousands of volunteer hours of assistance and comfort to people with AIDS and their loved ones. They developed and operated AIDS telephone crisis lines, provided advocacy, and in many cases conceived, printed, and distributed the first prevention and education material.

A special community was created by people who themselves were HIV-infected. The "People With AIDS" movement grew out of shared anger. Sick of being called AIDS victims, with heavy connotations of passivity and helplessness, these people fought actively to regain their health (Shilts, 1988). Tired of being called patients even when they were not in the hospital (Shilts), they mobilized, using insights gained from their personal struggles with AIDS, to contribute to the larger battle.

Implications for counseling. In order to work effectively with people with AIDS or at risk for AIDS, counselors will need to examine their own prejudices with respect to minority populations. How a counselor feels about gays, Blacks, Hispanics, intravenous drug users, and even hemophiliacs will influence his or her ability to understand and empathize with the client. Counselors working with PWAs or people at risk for AIDS will often have to work through the hurt and anger a client experiences as a result of societal hatred. Counselors will have to assure and reassure their clients that they will treat them differently than other people they may have encountered, that they will approach them with caring as opposed to condemnation.

An Emergent Trend in Education: "Just Say No"

Education plays the central role in the prevention of the AIDS crisis. Gallo and Montagnier (1988) wrote that, "even without a vaccine or a cure, what is already known could bring the epidemic under control" and that "there is a need for education about HIV infection—in clear, explicit language and as early as possible" (p. 48). Educational efforts of the 80s struggled with complex confounding issues of dogma and morality, and found it difficult, for the most part, to provide the cogent information that experts on AIDS called for. Instead, educational efforts in the 80s appropriated the catch phrase of the nation's drug prevention program and urged the American public to "just say no" to AIDS. How to say no, or what exactly to say no to, were disguised, disinfected, or altogether disregarded in educational programs and pamphlets.

Political forces may have influenced the minimalist approach to AIDS prevention. White House conservatives were convinced that AIDS education programs were cleverly designed covers to promote sodomy and sexual promiscuity (Shilts, 1988). An official Department of Education handbook, approved by the White House, urged teachers to stress "appropriate moral and social conduct" as the first line of defense against AIDS (Shilts). Many congressional efforts to forge bipartisan consensus on issues of research and education tended to fall apart on politically touchy issues like nondiscrimination hampered by ultraconservative Senator Jesse Helms's amendments decrying homosexuality.

A bright light in the field of education was embodied by Surgeon General C. Everett Koop. Koop, himself an ultraconservative fundamentalist, spent much of 1986 interviewing scientists, health officials, and gay community leaders. Out of those interviews he prepared the "Surgeon General's Report on Acquired Immune Deficiency Syndrome" and had tens of thousands of copies of the text printed and mailed to homes across the country. The report addressed, for one of the first times, the problem of AIDS in purely public health terms. Koop (1986) wrote that education should start at the earliest grade possible for children. He bluntly advocated widespread use of condoms and maintained that compulsory identification of virus carriers would be useless in fighting the disease.

Despite the surgeon general's report, by early 1987, the United States was still the only major industrialized nation that had not launched a coordinated education campaign against AIDS (Shilts, 1988). In contrast, European countries launched campaigns using billboards, newspaper advertisements, and television commercials urging people not to "die of ignorance" (Shilts).

Early educational efforts evolved within the gay community. Watson (1984) noted that gay men have been bombarded with more medical information than one person would normally receive in a lifetime. From the onset, the gay community in particular was challenged by the problem of developing preventive education about the need for moderating high-risk behaviors and adopting "safer sex" techniques (Martin & Vance, 1984).

Even with the best of intentions, the "just say no" approach to education was criticized as ineffective and misleading. Shernoff (1988) observed that highly visible and well-placed professionals provided unrealistic and unfounded advice regarding AIDS prevention. He offers former president of the American Association for Sex Educators, Counselors and Therapists, Teresa Crenshaw's statement that "the only absolutely safe sex is celibacy or masturbation" as an example. Shernoff maintained that although the statement is true in the abstract, it is unrealistic and irresponsible to expect people to either stop having sex or simply masturbate. Gochros (1988) corroborated this point, offering an astute quip by I. Reiss, professor at the University of Minnesota, who suggested that "vows of celibacy have a far higher breakage rate than condoms" (p. 255). Palacios-Jimenez and Shernoff (1988) found that when people ceased to abstain from sex after periods of "unwanted" celibacy, they were likely to engage in high-risk behavior. The "just say no" to sex campaign's greatest flaw lay in its inability to take into consideration the psychological functions sexual activities serve in many human beings. Gochros wrote that "by emphasizing the dangers of sex and ignoring the fact that most responsible sexual acts by most responsible people do not lead to pregnancy, disease, or death, the healthy, joyful naturalness of sexuality is obscured" (p. 256).

Educators often admonished entering into and maintaining a monogamous sexual relationship as the alternative to abstinence. This too is mistaken information; unless testing has established that both partners have not been exposed to HIV, there is little to ensure that a monogamous relationship is virus-free (Gochros, 1988). Advising clients to reduce their number of sex partners is, in and of itself, not helpful or even accurate (Shernoff, 1988). An individual who is the receptive partner in anal or vaginal intercourse with one seropositive person is at higher risk for becoming infected than a person who is involved in mutual masturbation with several different partners, regardless of their antibody status (Shernoff). Gochros critques other educational efforts to reduce the risk of AIDS in that they often treat sexual practices conforming to "safer sex" guidelines as second best.

Although in some of the most severely affected communities, sustained and intensive educational efforts were rewarded by striking changes in behavior, the gap between knowledge and personal action remained wide (Fineberg, 1988). In a national poll conducted in August 1987, more than 90% of Americans knew they could contract AIDS from having sex or sharing needles with an infected person. When asked about the possibility of contracting AIDS themselves, 90% of all respondents viewed their own risk as low or nonexistent (Fineberg). Fineberg wrote that "if the effectiveness of education is to be measured by behavioral change, success will not come easy" (p. 130). Gochros (1988) maintained that educators must deal with a cultural history in which condoms were seen as a symbol of immoral, clandestine, casual, and dirty sex. Furthermore, educators must assert that sexual desire, planned sexual encounters, sexual talk between actual or potential sexual partners, and condoms are good common sense.

Implications for counseling. Counseling is a form of educating, giving people new ways of seeing their world and new tools for interacting with it. Like a teacher who carefully reviews the curriculum of a class he or she will teach, counselors must examine the information on AIDS they will provide to their clients. Counselors must provide clients with clear, concise, and accurate information about AIDS and how it can be prevented.

An Emergent Trend in Counseling: Empowerment

If a single goal unifies all counselor orientations and approaches to treatment in the AIDS crisis, it is the goal of empowering those affected by AIDS. Empowerment demands that counselors and other human development specialists offer people the hope and tools needed to live a meaningful life in the face of a crisis.

Psychological effects of AIDS, both on the individual and on the collective psyche were slowly recognized in the 80s. Morin, Charles, and Malyon (1984) and Morin and Batchelor (1984) reported that whereas medical needs of people diagnosed with AIDS were being met, psychological needs were not. This is calamitous because AIDS patients are at high risk for psychological problems that are often underdiagnosed and undertreated (Perry & Tross, 1984).

Haney (1988), a social worker with AIDS, viewed many of the potential psychosocial consequences of AIDS as disconnections. AIDS disconnects people from the past, present, and future, from loved ones, from their ways of defining themselves such as job activities, capabilities, skills, and physical appearance, and, perhaps most importantly, from a sense of power and control over their life, hopes, dreams, and aspirations.

Goulden, Todd, and Hay (1984) suggested several steps in empowering clients with AIDS that center on the relief of depression. These steps included adopting stress-reducing activities, participating in support groups, channeling anger constructively, improving the quality of relationships, and avoiding the abuse of drugs and alcohol.

Counselors helping people with AIDS found they had to assist them to focus on learning to live with the illness. Haney (1988) offered six ways of providing empowerment to persons with AIDS. First, mental health professionals could help their clients focus on the positive, less fatalistic aspects of having AIDS. This is not to suggest denial but rather a reframing of the situation emphasizing how to make the most of an otherwise negative situation. Second, there is a healing power in hope and caring that the mental health worker must provide when others in the client's life are unable to supply this need. Third, mental health professionals could help people with AIDS reconnect with a support system. Fourth, mental health professionals could teach people with AIDS procedures to gain control of their illness and their lives. This could be accomplished in many different ways, from teaching creative visualization or guided meditation to offering anxiety and stress-reduction techniques. Fifth, mental health workers could help people with AIDS get rid of their victim mind-set. Finally, counselors can become advocates for the needs and rights of people with AIDS, standing by the belief in all people's worth and dignity.

Morin and Batchelor (1984) saw issues of loss and bereavement as important topics that must be addressed by people with AIDS, their lovers, and significant others. Baumgartner (1985) suggested that the healthy may need help in coping with "survivor's guilt," a constant wondering of why they survived accompanied by a fear of reinvesting themselves emotionally and sexually in new relationships. Lopez and Getzel (1984) recognized the existence of community mourning, also known as bereavement overload. Dr. James W. Dilly, executive director of the AIDS Health Project in San Francisco expressed fear that his city would be ill prepared for the "overload of grief" it would face as the AIDS death rate doubled, to six people a day by 1993 (Zonana & Morain, 1988).

Implications for counseling. Counselors working with people with AIDS and people at risk for AIDS will need to find ways to integrate into their practice techniques for empowering clients. Counselors will need to be prepared to confront grief reactions of immense intensity in their clients and in themselves. More than ever, counselors will need to find colleagues who can support and encourage their work.

AIDS in the Nineties: What Can Counselors Expect?

It is apparent from looking at the first decade of the AIDS crisis that the future will undoubtedly entail greater involvement on the part of counselors, educators, psychologists, social workers, nurses, and the world at large. Mann, Chin, Piot, and Quinn (1988) stated that although the AIDS pandemic is still in its early stages, it is apparent that AIDS is an unprecedented threat to global health. They see the global situation getting much worse before it can be brought under control.

Having examined the past, what projections can be made for the future of the AIDS crisis? Each day offers a change in the status of AIDS, whether that be in the realm of medicine, politics, social conditions, education, or counseling, making predicting the future a precarious task. Nonetheless, given the previously elaborated trends, it seems reasonable to suggest, at least tentatively, 10 areas for which counselors might prepare.

1. Counselors will see the number of AIDS cases continue to increase. Reports to the World Health Organization suggest that at least 5 million people worldwide are infected by the AIDS virus and that a million new cases of AIDS are likely by 1995 (Mann et al., 1988). Whether by working directly with people with AIDS, working with children whose parents have AIDS, or working with schools with HIV-infected students, counselors will inevitably find AIDS a part of their profession.

2. Counselors will face an increasing number of infected infants and children. Heyward and Curran (1988) indicated that children make up the fastest growing group of reported AIDS patients. In New York City in 1988, between 1% and 2% of all women giving birth were found to be infected with HIV (Fineberg, 1988). Most of these cases can be traced to intravenous drug use by the child's mother or her sexual partner. Counselors will have to develop new approaches to counseling these children in the coming decade.

3. Revisions will be needed in the nation's programs of providing health services. The AIDS epidemic will exacerbate the shortcomings in the system of paying for health care in the United States. In 1988, one in five AIDS patients had no insurance, 40% of AIDS patients were covered by Medicaid, which frequently paid less than the cost of care, and private insurers were often reluctant to cover the kinds of services most needed by people infected with HIV (Fineberg, 1988). Most private insurance is linked to employment, ensuring that at some point the prolonged illness of AIDS will result in the loss of insurance. Other major Western countries provide some sort of national health insurance, so that people struck with catastrophic illness do not find themselves scrambling to pay for basic care (Altman,

1986). Suggested ways of remedying the United States' problems in paying for health care include: state-based insurance risk pools or subsidies for uninsured patients, reliance on case managers to determine whether insurers should pay for services normally not covered, adjustments in the national standards of Medicaid eligibility and payment, simplification of the procedures for states to request flexibility in Medicaid coverage, further extension of insurance coverage for employees who lose their jobs, mandated employer health insurance, and broadened federal and state support of health insurance (Fineberg). If changes are not implemented and third-party reimbursement for mental health services is not available to people with HIV infections, low fee, community mental health clinics will be inundated with the burden of becoming the primary provider of treatment to people with AIDS.

4. Counselors will find increased attention placed on the plight of AIDS in Third World countries. In parts of Africa and the Caribbean, HIV infection is more prevalent than in the United States (Fineberg, 1988). Shilts (1988) reported a predominant feeling at the IV International AIDS Conference in Stockholm in 1988 that the true weight of the future AIDS epidemic would fall on the shoulders of health professionals in the Third World. Demographic projections suggest that the long-term impact of AIDS on Third World nations may be similar to that of a prolonged war (Fineberg). Gallo and Montagnier (1988) maintained that education alone will not stem the epidemic in some areas of the developing world and claimed that other measures will be necessary. Counselors will need to take a global perspective in their work with AIDS, networking with mental health professionals in Third World countries or offering to work in those countries themselves.

5. Counselors will be needed to minister to the inner city as it becomes plagued by the AIDS epidemic. For people in the inner city, a diagnosis of AIDS compounds the social stigma and low self-esteem they already experience as a result of their socioeconomic class. Numerous critical issues exist for HIV-infected residents of the inner city that will need to be addressed by counselors in the 1990s. Many people with AIDS in the inner city are IV drug users and therefore face a more rapid disease course than do non-IV drug users with AIDS (Marmor, 1984). Counselors will need to address the generally negative attitude toward IV drug users that has resulted in little professional support and few existing community resources (Honey, 1988).

Counselors will also have to contend with the lack of housing for people with AIDS in the inner city (Honey). Counselors will have to revise AIDS prevention education, which has frequently failed to take into account the cultural differences in sexual relationships among ethnic minority couples living in the inner city (Shernoff, 1988). Counselors will need to plan for long-term care of children if a parent with AIDS dies or is unable to care for the child. This task will be greatly compounded if the child is also infected, making placement in foster or adoptive homes extremely difficult (Honey).

6. Counselors will see AIDS become a significant legal issue. Given the current social and political climate of the nation, an increasing number of legal battles will be a part of the AIDS crisis of the 90s. Issues of quarantine are likely. The breach of confidentiality, already an issue in the late 80s (Gray & Harding, 1988; Kain, 1988), will be the basis for new legal rulings and legislation affecting the practice of psychotherapy and counseling.

7. Counselors will wait for scientists to develop new drugs and vaccines against the HIV. These scientists will, however, have to overcome shortfalls in funding and difficulties inherent in the HIV. Thomas (1988) wrote that a new class of antiviral drugs is needed, one capable of killing viruses inside the cells they invade without killing the cells themselves, but that the development of such pharmacological wonders is most difficult and unpredictable. Mathews and Bolognesi (1988) reported that the task of developing a vaccine is arduous in the face of one of the most intractable viral diseases in medical history, and pointed out four factors that make finding a vaccine for AIDS particularly difficult. First, ethical concerns abound because the only way to be sure a vaccine has warded off disease is to inject the vaccine recipient with HIV and observe the consequences. Second, clinicians expect to be confronted with a shortage of trial volunteers because healthy people may be reluctant to try a vaccine that has no demonstrated efficacy and because there simply may not be enough people in high-risk categories to provide statistically significant results. Third, recruitment problems will only worsen as more vaccines are developed, each requiring thousands of people for testing. Finally, uncertainty surrounding the risks and liability of vaccine-related injuries and compensation for them could ultimately hinder vaccine development. Given these difficulties, "avoiding" AIDS by placing all hope on a cure will not be a realisitic option for counselors or their clients; instead both will be forced to confront the excruciatingly painful issues that loom in the days ahead.

8. New counselors and other health professionals will be needed to take the place of health professionals exhausted and depleted by their work with the epidemic. Fineberg (1988) reported that fewer physicians today are choosing to pursue careers in internal medicine, suggesting that AIDS may be part of the reason. Simmons-Alling (1984) characterized four ways in which mental health professionals are affected by working with HIV-infected clients: A-anxiety, I-isolation, D-drain, and S-stress, any of which can lead to professional burnout. Dr. Joel Weisman, who co-reported the first cases of AIDS in Los Angeles in June 1980, feels that there is an "avoidance phenomenon" among health professionals and that "while in an ideal world, every physician should treat the patient with AIDS, in the real world, that's just not going to happen" (Simross, 1988). The counseling profession will need to counter its own trend toward avoidance with involvement. Counselors will need to find ways to work with people afraid of AIDS, at risk for AIDS, or ill with AIDS, so as to minimize their own emotional burnout.

9. Hospice will become more recognized as a preferred way of caring for people with AIDS. The use of an interdisciplinary team approach to working with people dying of AIDS greatly benefits both the person with AIDS and the team members. Counselors will find themselves included in these teams along with physicians, nurses, pastoral care persons, and trained volunteers. Additionally, because hospice care is often offered in the patient's home or in special supportive care environments, clients will no longer be able to come to counselors' offices. Counselors will have to go to their clients.

10. Compassion will be greatly needed. In the face of the escalating tragedy of AIDS that affronts the world in the decade of the 1990s, it will be important for counselors and others to find the human side to the crisis. Compassion may, more than anything, be the crucial determinant of the future of the AIDS epidemic.

Summary and Conclusion

Much can be written about the first decade of the AIDS crisis and certainly much more will be written. This chapter examined five major areas affected by the major health crisis of the 80s and quite possibly that of the 90s. Medicine, politics, society, education, and counseling have all, in one way or another, been called upon to meet the challenge of AIDS. In the last 10 years many trends have appeared: new words, new political battles, new forms of old prejudice, new lessons to be learned, and a new class of clients needing help. Each of these trends has affected the field of counseling. The next 10 years will undoubtedly bring many more trends; 10 such future trends were mentioned in the course of this chapter. Crucial to the future of AIDS is how we, as counselors, respond to the calls for help we receive. In the face of whatever frustration, resentment, anxiety, or stress we may encounter, can we open our hearts and offer those suffering from the effects of AIDS our intelligence, our integrity, our selflessness and our compassion? I hope our answer to this question is affirmative. The importance of our answer is captured by His Holiness Tenzin Gaytso, the Fourteenth Dali Lama when he says, "Out of my experience, I tell my friends wherever I go about the importance of love and compassion. Deep down we must have real affection for each other, a clear realization or recognition of our shared human status."

References

Altman, D. (1986). AIDS in the mind of America. New York: Doubleday.

American Foundation for AIDS Research. (1988). *AIDS/HIV experimental treatment directory*. New York: Author.

Baumgartner, G.H. (1985). *AIDS: Psychosocial factors in the acquired immune deficiency syndrome*. Springfield, IL: Charles C Thomas.

Fineberg, H.V. (1988). The social dimensions of AIDS. *Scientific American, 4*, 128–134.

Gallo, R.C., & Montagnier, L. (1988). AIDS in 1988. *Scientific American, 4*, 40–51.

Gochros, H.L. (1988). Risks of abstinence: Sexual decision making in the AIDS era. *Social Work, 3*, 254–256.

Goulden, T., Todd, R., & Hay, R. (1984). AIDS and community supportive services: Understanding and management of psychosocial needs. *Medical Journal of Australia, 27*, 582–586.

Gray, L.A., & Harding, A.K. (1988). Confidentiality limits with clients who have the AIDS virus. *Journal of Counseling and Development, 66*, 219–223.

Haney, P. (1988). Providing empowerment to the person with AIDS. *Social Work, 33*, 251–253.

Heyward, W.L. & Curran, J.W. (1988). The epidemiology of the AIDS virus. *Scientific American, 4,* 72–81.

Honey, E. (1988). AIDS and the inner city: Critical issues. *Social Casework, 69,* 365–370.

Kagay, M.R. (1988, October 14). Survey finds little sympathy for gays or addicts with AIDS. *Los Angeles Herald Examiner,* pp. 1, 8.

Kain, C.D. (1988). To breach or not to breach: Is that the question? A response to Gray and Harding. *Journal of Counseling and Development, 66,* 224–225.

Koop, C.E. (1986). *The Surgeon General's report on acquired immunodeficiency syndrome.* Washington, DC: U.S. Public Health Services.

Leary, W.E. (1988, October 20). FDA plans to approve new drugs faster. *Los Angeles Herald Examiner,* p. 3.

Leibowitch, J. (1985). *A strange virus of unknown origin.* New York: Ballentine Books.

Lopez, D.J., & Getzel, G.S. (1984). Helping gay AIDS patients in crisis. *Social Casework,* September, 387–394.

Mann, J.M., Chin, J., Piot, P., & Quinn, T. (1988). The international epidemiology of AIDS. *Scientific American, 4,* 82–89.

Marmor, M. (1984). The epidemic of Acquired Immunodeficiency Syndrome (AIDS) and suggestions for its control in drug abusers. *Journal of Substance Abuse and Treatment, 1,* 237–247.

Martin, J.L., & Vance, C.S. (1984). Behavioral and psychosocial factors in AIDS: Methodological and substantive issues. *American Psychologist, 11,* 1303–1308.

Mathews, T.J., & Bolognesi, D.P. (1988). AIDS vaccines. *Scientific American, 4,* 120–127.

Molotsky, I. (1988, October 14). Congressional compromise gets major AIDS bill through. *Los Angeles Herald Examiner,* p. 8.

Monette, P. (1988). *Borrowed time: An AIDS memoir.* New York: Harcourt Brace Jovanovich.

Morin, S.F., & Batchelor, W. (1984). Responding to the psychological crises of AIDS. *Public Health Reports, 99,* 4–9.

Morin, S.F., Charles, K.A., & Malyon, A.K. (1984). The psychological impact of AIDS on gay men. *American Psychologist, 11,* 1288–1293.

Osborn, J.E. (1987). The AIDS epidemic: Discovery of a new disease. In H.L. Dalton & S. Burris (Eds.), *AIDS and the law: A guide for the public* (pp. 17–27). New Haven, CT: Yale Press.

Palacios-Jimenez, L., & Shernoff, M. (1988). AIDS: Prevention is the only vaccine available . . . an AIDS prevention education model. *Journal of Social Work and Human Sexuality, 6,* 27–34.

Perry, S.W., & Tross, S. (1984). Psychiatric problems of AIDS patients at the New York Hospital: Preliminary report. *Public Health Report, 2,* 200–205.

Schram, N.R. (1988, September 7). The short history of a long tragedy. *Los Angeles Herald Examiner,* pp. 1, 4.

Shernoff, M. (1988). Integrating safer-sex counseling into social work practice. *Social Casework, 69,* 365–370.

Shilts, R. (1988). *And the band played on: Politics, people, and the AIDS epidemic.* New York: Penguin Books.

Simon, R. (Ed.). (1988). Confronting the specter of AIDS: What do therapists have to offer? *The Family Therapy Networker, 12*(1).

Simmons-Alling, S. (1984). AIDS: Psychosocial needs of the health care worker. *Topics in Clinical Nursing, 7,* 31–37.

Simross, L. (1988, July 27). The unwanted challenge. *Los Angeles Times,* pp. 1, 3.

Stulberg, I., & Smith, M. (1988). Psychosocial impact of the AIDS epidemic on the lives of gay men. *Social Work, 33,* 277–281.

Thomas, L. (1988). AIDS: An unknown distance still to go. *Scientific American, 4,* 152.

Watson, L. (1984, Oct.). Living with AIDS. *Medical Journal of Australia, 27,* 559–560.

Yarchoan, R., Hiroaki, M., & Broder, S. (1988). AIDS therapies. *Scientific American, 4,* 110–119.

Zonana, V.F., & Morain, D. (1988, May 12). AIDS toll in S.F.: City under siege. *Los Angeles Times,* pp. 1, 3, 18.

Chapter 2

A RESEARCH UPDATE FOR COUNSELORS

Joseph R. Guydish and Maria Ekstrand

A child in your school district has been diagnosed with AIDS. The parents are distraught, one teacher has refused to have the child in class, parents of other children do not yet know, and the child understands only that he is scared and sick. When the principal phones to set a meeting, you mark the anxiety in her voice.

A physician refers a young woman with AIDS. Infected by her bisexual ex-husband, she was sick for months before the diagnosis was made. AIDS was unexpected in a heterosexual woman with no history of intravenous (IV) drug use. Ridden by fatigue and nausea, she is no longer able to work or adequately care for her two young children. After being in therapy for several months, she dies.

These are scenarios of AIDS in America. To those already initiated they represent scenarios of today, and for the uninitiated they are scenarios of tomorrow. Counselors have a pivotal and expanding role in responding to the AIDS epidemic. The goal of this chapter is to provide counselors with a survey of current and clinically focused HIV-related research. After a brief review of HIV epidemiology, our discussion is organized

This chapter was supported by the National Institutes of Mental Health and Drug Abuse through the Center for AIDS Prevention Studies, University of California, San Francisco (grant 1P50 MH42459).

in terms of those at risk of infection, those who are seropositive but asymptomatic, and those who are diagnosed with AIDS or ARC. Our central theme is prevention, which continues to hold the greatest hope for slowing the spread of HIV and minimizing the associated human suffering and loss of life.

Current Epidemiology

It is now over 8 years since the initial and foreboding reports of pneumocystis carinii pneumonia (PCP) and Kaposi's sarcoma (KS) among homosexual men appeared (Centers for Disease Control, 1981a; CDC, 1981b). The World Health Organization (WHO) reported nearly 112,000 AIDS cases in 140 countries as of August 1988 (CDC, 1988a). Worldwide reporting is incomplete, however, due to inadequate health care and AIDS diagnostic facilities in some areas, and because some governments were slow to acknowledge the presence of AIDS in their country (Piot, Plummer, Mhalu, Lamboray, Chin, & Mann, 1988). Consequently, the WHO estimates 250,000 to 300,000 AIDS cases globally, and 5 to 10 million people infected with HIV (CDC, 1988a; 1988b).

In the United States specifically, the Centers for Disease Control reported a cumulative total of over 76,000 cases in October 1988 (CDC, 1988c). Most adult U.S. AIDS cases (88%) are among gay and bisexual men or IV drug users, 4% among non-IV drug using heterosexuals, and the remaining cases are related to hemophilia, blood transfusion, or are undetermined (CDC, 1988c). Because the case count increases substantially each week, future projections communicate more effectively the magnitude of the epidemic. By 1992, 365,000 U.S. AIDS patients will have been diagnosed, of whom 263,000 will have died. Currently, 1 to 1.5 million people in the United States are thought to be infected with HIV (CDC, 1988d). The magnitude of the epidemic now, coupled with its projected growth, necessitates that counselors be well informed about AIDS.

Persons at Risk

HIV is now well entrenched in the United States, and everyone is at some risk of infection. Individuals most in danger of HIV infection, however, are at risk because they engage in behaviors that facilitate viral transmission, primarily unprotected anal and vaginal intercourse and IV drug use. Researchers often use the term "HIV spectrum disease" to reflect the growing awareness that the many manifestations of HIV infection are symptomatic of the same immunologic dysfunction. Specifically, the distinction between AIDS and ARC has come under fire because it applies different diagnoses where there is no difference in the underlying causal agent (HIV), or the underlying disease process. Although current knowledge about HIV spectrum disease is organized by risk groups, and although risk group generalizations are useful in planning and targeting interventions, risk of infection is determined by individual behavior.

It now seems that nearly all persons infected with HIV will eventually develop AIDS (Lui, Darrow, & Rutherford, 1988; Lemp et al., 1988), a disease that remains both incurable and fatal. Consequently, the central issue in working with persons at risk is the prevention of infection by changing risk-related behaviors. In the sections below we discuss a theoretical model of health behavior change, followed by recent HIV-related prevention literature organized by groups at risk.

The Health Belief Model of Risk Reduction

A modified version of the health belief model (HBM) provides a theoretical framework for studying risk behaviors, designing risk reduction interventions, and counseling individuals for behavior change. Based on the classic Health Belief Model (Becker, 1974), the modified version also incorporates self-efficacy theory (Bandura, 1986) and the importance of perceived peer and social norms. The role of self-efficacy in health behavior has gained increasing recognition, and this construct was recently incorporated into the classic HBM (Rosenstock, Strecher, & Becker, 1988).

The HBM assumes that beliefs are major determinants of behavior, and several types of beliefs are thought to influence preventive health action: (1) knowledge of the disease and of preventive behavior; (2) perceived susceptibility to a given disease and beliefs regarding the severity of the consequences; (3) the perceived benefits and costs of engaging in preventive behavior; (4) a cue to action that triggers preventive behavior, such as the illness of a friend or reading about the disease; (5) peer and social norms, which may be perceived as supporting or discouraging preventive behavior; and (6) a sense of self-efficacy, or seeing oneself as capable of engaging in preventive behavior.

Effective HIV prevention strategies typically address multiple aspects of the health belief model, such as enhancing self-efficacy or intervening to change community norms, in addition to increasing knowledge. We will return to the HBM at the end of this chapter to further discuss its application to the problems of changing risk behavior.

Risk Reduction Among Gay Men

Gay men in San Francisco have made significant and lasting risk behavior changes in response to AIDS. Several reports document reductions in the number of sexual partners and frequency of unprotected insertive and receptive anal intercourse, both firmly established high-risk behaviors for the transmission of HIV (Friedland & Klein, 1987).

The San Francisco City Clinic Cohort Study was initiated in 1978 to examine hepatitis B among men seeking treatment in a sexually transmitted disease (STD) clinic. A subsample (n = 125) of the original cohort was followed longitudinally to better understand the effects of HIV infection. Drastic behavior changes were reported in this sample by 1985, with 90% of participants reducing the number of partners from a median of 16 to a median 1 (Doll, Darrow, O'Malley, Bodecker, & Jaffee, 1987).

A longitudinal study of single men in the area of San Francisco hardest hit by the AIDS epidemic (San Francisco Men's Health Study) helped identify sexual behaviors associated with increased risk of infection and demonstrated significant reductions in the practice of these behaviors (Winkelstein et al., 1987a). In contrast to many types of behavior change, the reported reductions in sexual risk behavior are remarkably stable. Fewer than 6% of the gay and bisexual participants reported any recidivism following initial risk reduction (Ekstrand & Coates, 1988). Changes of this magnitude and stability are unprecedented in health behaviors (Coates, Stall, & Hoff, 1988), and laboratory data in this sample bear out self-reported behavior change; the incidence of new infection is less than 1% per year (Winkelstein et al., 1987b).

Behavior change among gay and bisexual men is not limited to San Francisco. Martin (1987) studied 745 gay men in New York between 1981 and 1985. In this cohort 40% reported some change toward safer sexual practices, including a 72% reduction in number of partners. Similarly, the percent of participants in monogamous relationships increased from 8% to 14% during the study period. Other studies suggest that behavior change has occurred in gay communities outside of these AIDS epicenters, although the magnitude of change reported is usually less dramatic.

Predictors of risk reduction include being older, agreeing with health guidelines, and having a sense of personal efficacy. In contrast, the use of alcohol and drugs, denial, and the belief that one has been exposed to HIV but successfully "fought it off" have been associated with high-risk behaviors (Ekstrand & Coates, 1988; Stall, McKusick, Wiley, Coates, & Ostrow, 1986). Gay men at higher risk of infection may also be less open about their homosexuality, less likely to be members of gay organizations, have less satisfying social networks, and experience an absence of supportive norms compared with low-risk gay men (Joseph, Montgomery, Kessler, Ostrow, & Wortmen, 1988).

Several authors have discussed the "San Francisco Model" in explaining risk reduction among gay men in this city (Coates & Greenblatt, in press; Catania, Coates, Kegeles, Ekstrand, Guydish, & Bye, 1988). Prevention efforts in San Francisco have relied heavily on community-based approaches and volunteer organizations to change social norms related to sexual practices, and to encourage safe sex as an acceptable alternative to high-risk practices. One well-known community-based risk reduction program in San Francisco is STOP AIDS (Puckett & Bye, 1987), which uses small group formats to encourage risk reduction among gay men. Important components of this program include opportunities for participants to clarify thoughts and feelings about AIDS and its impact on the gay community, learn how others have adapted to the epidemic, share feelings about safe and unsafe sex, and express views about AIDS prevention needs that are then relayed to community leaders and organizations.

The results of the STOP AIDS program indicate that participants have a greater sense of personal responsibility for ending the AIDS epidemic, that there is considerable support for the practice of safer sex in the gay and bisexual community, and that most participants can make a commitment to practice safe sex.

These findings have implications for counselors' prevention efforts. It is essential to target younger gay men, and particularly those not yet integrated into gay networks and organizations. These campaigns may be more successful if, in addition to health education, they assist participants in building social support, include social skills training components, and discourage having sex under the influence of alcohol and other drugs.

Risk Reduction Among Substance Abusers

Substance abuse is a linchpin in the continuing HIV epidemic. IV drug users represent 19% of U.S. AIDS cases reported through October 1988, with an additional 7% reported among gay men who also use IV drugs. Moreover, the proportion of AIDS cases each year having IV drug use as the only risk factor increased from 16% in 1987 to 23% in 1988 (CDC, 1988c). The spread of infection among IV users can be explosive, and HIV seroprevalence in some IV drug user samples is over 50% (Des Jarlais & Friedman, 1987).

Risk is not limited to needle users themselves, as 60% of heterosexually transmitted AIDS cases and over half of pediatric cases are among heterosexual partners and children of IV users (see Des Jarlais, Friedman, Casriel, & Kott, 1987). The secondary spread of HIV to sexual partners and children prompted one author to identify IV drug use as "the real heterosexual epidemic" (Moss, 1987, p. 389). The secondary spread of HIV related to IV drug use is also a Black and Hispanic epidemic. Of all heterosexual AIDS cases associated with IV drug use in the United States, 80% occurred in these two ethnic groups (Selik, Castro, & Pappaioanou, 1988).

The abuse of substances through non-IV routes is also associated with HIV infection. Substance abusing individuals may trade sex for drugs, use stimulant drugs to enhance sexual desire, or use hypnotics to decrease sexual inhibition (Clark & Washburn, 1988). Sexual activity occurring under drug influence is less likely to be safe sex (Stall et al., 1986), and the level of alcohol consumption is positively associated with high-risk sexual behavior in heterosexual as well as gay and bisexual men in San Francisco (Guydish, Coates, & Ekstrand, 1988; Ekstrand & Coates, 1988). The use of crack cocaine in particular, now endemic among youth in some urban centers, may significantly increase risk of HIV infection. In one ethnographic study crack users reported higher numbers of sexual partners, more frequent infection with other STDs, and infrequent condom use, despite adequate knowledge about HIV transmission (Bowser, 1988). Finally, some drugs have immunosuppressive effects (Hubbard, Marsden, Cavanaugh, Rachal, & Ginzburg, 1988), and may facilitate infection or negatively affect the course of illness.

Successful prevention in segments of urban gay populations has come mainly from grass-roots efforts wherein specific gay communities mobilized political, financial, and educational resources necessary to stem the spread of the virus. Substance abusing populations, by contrast, typically lack the networks and resources to mobilize equivalent grass-roots efforts. Consequently, prevention among substance abusers is largely an effort of health care providers, public health professionals, and recovering addicts. Substance abuse treatment programs, because of their familiarity and acceptance by drug users, are likely centers for AIDS prevention. Sustained HIV prevention efforts conducted in drug treatment programs may reach beyond clients themselves to partners and families of users in treatment, and may have a secondary or ripple effect among users not in treatment (Bixler, Palacios-Jimenez, & Springer, 1987).

Although the discontinuation of drug use is the most desirable goal, effective prevention must include other strategies. Sorensen, Gibson, Heitzmann, Dumontet, & Acampora (1988) presented a conceptual framework for HIV prevention among substance abusers that includes four levels of individual protection. The strongest defense, and the one providing the best insurance against infection for IV drug users, is to stop drug use. A second but weaker defense is to stop using drugs through the intravenous route. The third level, for those who continue IV drug use, is to avoid sharing needles. For those who continue to share needles, the last defense is disinfecting needles with bleach prior to each injection.

Practitioners and researchers are deploying innovative prevention strategies consistent with these levels of defense, and are using multiple points of entry into the substance abusing

community. At one end of the spectrum, treatment programs
are training clients in risk reduction practices (Sorensen et al.,
1988), and conducting clinic-based outreach to IV drug users
and their sexual partners (Gibson, Wermuth, Lovelle-Drache,
Ergas, & Sorensen, 1988; Wermuth, Ham, & Gibson, 1988). At
the opposite end of the spectrum, street outreach workers are
delivering information and strategies to active addicts who may
not want treatment at this time (Watters, 1987).

Risk Reduction Among Adolescents

Adolescents have a high prevalence of many behaviors related to HIV acquisition and transmission. A large proportion
(50%–70%) of adolescents are sexually active, with a marked
increase from 1971–1979 among 15–19-year-olds (Zelnik &
Kantner, 1980; Harris, 1981). In addition, adolescents report
very little condom use. Kegeles, Adler, and Irwin (1988) surveyed 325 sexually active teenagers over a 1-year period and
found that although adolescents perceived condom use as preventing STDs and placed a high value on prevention, consistent
condom use remained poor at the 1-year follow up (only 2%
of women and 8% of men reported always using condoms).

That more adolescents are sexually active but few use condoms is supported by increasing rates of STDs in this age group.
Approximately 50% of all STD cases occur in individuals under
25 years of age, and rates decrease exponentially with increasing
age (NIAID, 1980; Bell & Holmes, 1984). Strunin and Hingson
(1987) surveyed Massachusetts adolescents and found that of
the 70% who were sexually active, only 15% had changed their
behavior to reduce AIDS risk. Of those, only 20% used effective
methods. Consequently, only 2% of adolescents in this sample
engaged in effective HIV-preventive behaviors.

The latency between HIV infection and symptom development is so long that many of those infected as adolescents
will not get sick until the early 20s, at the age where 20% of
AIDS cases presently occur. Consistent with their level of cognitive development, many adolescents have a sense of immor-
tality (Elkind, 1967), and are less likely to feel susceptible to
HIV infection. Accordingly, many teenagers may find it difficult to engage in HIV-related preventive behaviors. Moreover,
basic knowledge of AIDS and preventive behaviors among adolescents is highly variable and riddled with misperceptions

(DiClemente, Zorn, & Temoshok, 1986). For example, most students in this study knew that gay men are at increased risk of acquiring AIDS, but also believed lesbian women to be at high risk. Of all teenagers, minority adolescents seem to have the highest risk of infection. Fullilove and Fullilove (1987) found that minority adolescents initiate sexual activity earlier, report a more erratic use of contraceptive practices, have a greater likelihood of contracting STDs and becoming pregnant, delay treatment longer, and have less sexual education knowledge than White adolescents.

In summary, many sexually active adolescents currently seem to lack the knowledge, health beliefs, and probably also the skills needed for risk reduction. In order to be effective, prevention campaigns targeting this age group need to take the unique characteristics of adolescents into account.

Risk Reduction in the General Population

AIDS is a sexually transmitted disease. Data from partner studies, where sexual transmission from infected individuals to their heterosexual partners is studied, clearly demonstrate bi-directional transmission. In studies evaluating male to female transmission the proportion of infected partners ranges from 9% to 60%, and for female to male transmission it ranges from 0% to 100% (Padian, 1987). Those studies reporting the highest percentages included index partners from Haiti and Africa where, unlike in the United States, heterosexual transmission is a primary vector for the spread of HIV.

Several population-based studies indicate differences in the prevalence of HIV infection. Among blood donors, a population where seropositive individuals usually self-select out, about 1 in 5,000 tests positive (CDC, 1987). Among applicants for military service the prevalence is about 1 in 700 (Burke et al, 1987). Among patients admitted to six sentinel hospitals, inmates in the Federal Bureau of Prisons, and Job Corps entrants the prevalence is about 1 in 300 (CDC, 1988d).

Not all of those infected are in traditional "high-risk groups." The CDC currently estimates that 80,000 to 160,000 non-IV drug using heterosexuals are infected in the United States (CDC, 1988e). Moreover, as the pool of infected heterosexuals increases, the incidence of heterosexual infection is also likely to increase. Factors potentially associated with heterosexual infection risk include number of sexual partners (CDC, 1988f), drug use (Goldsmith, 1988), other sexually transmitted diseases (Simonsen et al., 1988), and heterosexual anal intercourse (Bolling & Voeller, 1987).

The heterosexual spread of AIDS is not expected to reach widespread and epidemic proportions (CDC, 1988d). Instead, heterosexual AIDS will probably develop in a pattern more similar to that of other STDs, where pockets of individuals who continue to engage in high-risk behaviors will become infected (Padian, 1987). From a public health viewpoint, however, any spread of a fatal but preventable disease is unacceptable.

Regarding heterosexual prevention, Hearst and Hulley (1988) suggested that knowledge of one's sexual partner prior to engaging in unprotected intercourse constitutes the most important precaution. This strategy assumes a rational, cautious, and time-consuming process of selecting sexual partners, a process not always practiced. It also implies, wrongly, that one can avoid infection by identifying safe partners rather than by practicing safe behaviors. Haverkos and Edelman (1988) advocated more conservative prevention strategies that include making all sexually active individuals aware of HIV infection risk, and reducing the number of sexual partners. Furthermore, during any sexual activity with **possibly** infected persons, contact with semen, vaginal secretions, and other fluids that may contain HIV should be avoided (Haverkos & Edelman). The emphasis here is on the practice of safe sexual behaviors, and the implication is that nearly all partners are "possibly" infected. Specifically, sexually active adults who are not involved in a long-standing monogamous relationship, or in a monogamous relationship where both partners have tested seronegative, are possibly infected.

Asymptomatic Seropositives

The discovery of HIV in 1983 and the availability of antibody testing in 1985 brought a new and difficult question: "Should I be tested?" Initially, many physicians and mental health professionals counseled against testing because (1) treatment for asymptomatic seropositives was not available, and (2) the knowledge of a positive test result could create significant stress that may itself contribute to immunocompromise. However, with the continuing spread of the epidemic, the expansion of knowledge about HIV, and the development of prophylactic treatments, testing is now strongly advocated by some (Redfield & Burke, 1988).

The mean incubation period of HIV, from infection to diagnosis, is variously estimated at 5 years, 7.8 years, and most recently at 11 years (Lemp et al., 1988). Significant individual and public health benefits may be realized in this time period if a person is aware of his or her seropositive status. Individual advantages include the possibility of slowing disease progression by preventing reinfection and by preventive treatment and health maintenance. Public health advantages include the opportunity to slow the spread of HIV by preventing infection of others. The individual costs of testing, of living with the knowledge of HIV infection, are also great. Working with seropositive individuals is discussed in a later chapter. Our focus here is limited to the role of antibody testing in risk behavior change, and the psychological and emotional impact of a positive test result.

The Role of Antibody Testing

In November 1984, 69% of all gay men participating in the AIDS Behavioral Research Project (N = 560) were interested in being tested once an antibody test was developed (Coates, Morin, & McKusick, 1987). In a follow-up study, after antibody testing became available, only 6% of this cohort had been tested and an additional 9% planned to be tested. Reasons cited for not having been tested included ambiguity regarding the meaning of a positive test result, lack of treatments for HIV infection, and confidentiality. The AIDS Behavioral Research Project also examined the behavioral and psychological consequences of testing. Those who were antibody positive showed significantly greater reductions in high-risk behaviors than both the negative and untested subjects. Ten seropositives reported still engaging in high-risk behaviors. Of the 10, 8 believed they had been exposed to HIV but that their bodies had successfully fought off the virus. A common motivation for testing was to find out whether one was capable of transmitting the virus. The authors point out that this has implications for public education programs, which might profitably focus on the desire to protect others as well as oneself. Antibody testing also had mental health consequences, with seropositive men reporting increased levels of stress and depression, as well as an increase in relationship problems following testing.

Fox, Odaka, Brookmeyer, and Polk (1987) studied 1,001 gay and bisexual men in the Washington/Baltimore area in 1984– 86. In this study 67% of men chose to learn their serostatus, and all of these men showed a decline in high-risk activity over the 18-month follow-up. However, a positive test result led to greater behavior change than did a negative one.

In a similar study, 270 homosexual men were surveyed at a Boston community health center (McCusker, Stoddard, Mayer, Zapka, Morrison, & Saltzman, 1988). Seropositive men who were informed of their results reduced the frequency of un- protected insertive anal intercourse more than did seronegative men. These participants also reported psychological conse- quences of knowing that they were seropositive. Specifically, they reported both depression (94%) and anger (49%) much more frequently than did the seropositives who were unaware of their status (65% and 0% respectively).

The above findings are remarkably consistent. Testing and counseling among gay men seems to produce behavior change, particularly for seropositive individuals. This risk reduction has a cost, however: Seropositive individuals report increased psy- chological distress upon discovering their antibody status. This finding underscores the importance of counseling, with appro- priate referrals to more extensive mental health services when needed, in combination with anonymous HIV testing.

These studies also highlight the dramatic emotional impact of HIV spectrum disease, as even asymptomatic individuals experience psychological distress on receiving a positive HIV test result. As patients later develop physical symptoms and ultimately receive an AIDS diagnosis, distress is likely to be a prominent and consistent emotional feature of the disease. One study reported a higher suicide rate for people with AIDS than for the general population, and higher than that for patients with Huntington's disease or cancer (Marzuk et al., 1988). This study was later criticized on methodological grounds (Beltan- gady, 1988), and further research is needed to clarify the re- lationship of HIV spectrum disease to suicide. In working with HIV-affected patients, the counselor should evaluate suicide potential as when working with other depressed, chronically ill, crisis, or dying patients.

Persons With AIDS and ARC

Central issues in working with people with AIDS/ARC (PWAs) include efforts to slow disease progression, enhance quality of life, and prevent infection of others. Although there are multiple and significant psychosocial issues in working with PWAs (Dilley, Ochitill, Perl, & Volberding, 1985), our discussion is limited to the biopsychosocial model, the psychological impact of an AIDS or ARC diagnosis, and the role of co-factors.

Biologically, AIDS is an immunoregulatory disease characterized by progressive deterioration of immune responsiveness, leaving the host open to a horrifying array of opportunistic infections that eventually result in death. Psychologically, AIDS may be characterized as a terminal illness or as a chronic debilitating illness, with all of the associated trauma, grief, and loss. Because AIDS continues to affect previously stigmatized segments of our society (gay men, IV drug users, and minorities), and because it is a costly and frightening disease, issues of prejudice and discrimination are boldly prominent.

For reasons such as these, AIDS and ARC require a biopsychosocial perspective that considers interactions of biological, emotional, behavioral, and cultural factors (Solomon & Temoshok, 1987). Although there is little experimental evidence that the course of HIV spectrum disease is affected by psychosocial factors, the more general relationship between stress and immunosuppression is now well accepted (e.g., Solomon, 1985). With respect to AIDS, repeated immunologic mobilization in response to biologic or psychosocial insult may activate latent HIV (Solomon & Temoshok) or further weaken an already embattled immune system. Continued IV drug use among seropositive individuals, for example, is associated with the rate of decline of T4 cells (Des Jarlais, Friedman, Marmor et al., 1987). Consequently, it is vital in the treatment of PWAs to consider behavioral, psychological, and social support factors that may bolster or maintain immunocompetence.

One such factor is the stress associated with the diagnosis itself. In a number of studies AIDS and ARC patients were compared with patients having more socially acceptable illnesses, such as chronic renal failure or bone marrow transplants, and with healthy controls. A diagnosis of AIDS or ARC often creates unique psychological problems not encountered by other terminally ill patients. AIDS and ARC patients reported increased levels of anger and tension in response to their diagnosis. Many showed high levels of anxiety, depression, confusion, and bewilderment, possibly related to the uncertainty surrounding this disease. These patients were also more likely to express fears of social abandonment and isolation than the non-HIV terminally ill patients. Furthermore, many patients reported feelings of guilt and self-blame, sometimes seeing their illness as a form of punishment. The authors attribute these findings to the fact that AIDS is primarily a disease of those already shut out by mainstream society, and the fears of the general population that AIDS might be casually transmitted (Donlou, Wolcott, Gottlieb, & Landsverk, 1985; Nichols, 1985; Holland & Tross, 1985).

Several co-factors also are thought to affect immunocompetence, either by enabling transmission of HIV or by altering disease progression. HIV infection may be facilitated by genital ulcers, including those resulting from STDs such as chlamydia and herpes simplex virus 2 (Greenblatt, Lukehart, & Plummer, 1988). Similarly, the use of oral contraceptives is associated with an increased likelihood of infection among women (Plummer et al., 1988). Though the mechanism underlying this relationship is not known, oral contraceptives may change the composition of cervical mucus in a way that facilitates infection. Other possible co-factors include the number of sexual partners, engaging in receptive anal intercourse, and the lack of circumcision.

The most consistent factor for disease progression is duration of HIV infection, so that the longer a person has been infected the greater the likelihood of having disease symptoms (Jason, Lui, Ragni, Darrow, & Hessol, 1988). This robust relationship has been found in separate studies of the same population, as well as in studies comparing different populations. There have been fewer bahavioral co-factors identified for disease progression than for infection. Hessol et al. (1988) examined the association between demographic, behavioral, and medical variables and the likelihood of developing AIDS. Using a multivariate analysis and controlling for duration of infection, the use of certain drugs (such as hallucinogens) and infection with other STDs (such as gonnorhea) were both associated with progression to AIDS.

The importance of co-factors in HIV spectrum disease is a matter of some contention, and the available data do not conclusively establish these variables as true biologic co-factors.

However, these studies clearly suggest that PWAs should avoid repeated infection with HIV, avoid contracting STDs (by using condoms and reducing the number of sexual partners), and reduce or eliminate intake of alcohol and illicit drugs.

Implications for Counselors

As the epidemic continues to grow, extending beyond current geographic and risk group boundaries, counselors will be increasingly called upon to meet the myriad psychosocial challenges of HIV spectrum disease. On the near horizon there is neither cure nor vaccine, and the current most effective means of slowing the epidemic is prevention. This means preventing noninfected persons from becoming infected, preventing infected persons from infecting others and, for those who are symptomatic, slowing disease progression by attending to physical and emotional health needs.

The implementation of preventive interventions, targeting specific groups defined by age, ethnicity, or type of risk behavior, may minimize HIV infection among those at risk. Early identification of positive serostatus, close medical monitoring, and preventive health care are indicated for asymptomatic seropositives. For persons with AIDS or ARC, life-style modifications, enhancement of social support, avoidance of co-factors, and amelioration of the many psychosocial stressors attendant to disease are likely to improve both quality and duration of life. For all persons with HIV spectrum disease, preventing the infection of others is a paramount public health concern.

In helping individuals make those behavioral changes requisite to effective HIV prevention, the modified health belief model points to the importance of assessing HIV-related beliefs. Because knowledge alone is not a good predictor of preventive behavior, simply educating clients is not likely to lead to behavior change. Rather, the counselor should assess client beliefs using the framework of the HBM. Do seronegative clients see themselves as susceptible to AIDS or HIV infection or do they see themselves as somehow immune? Do seropositive clients believe they are capable of infecting others, or do they believe that they have a "less infectious strain" of the virus? Do they perceive AIDS as fatal, or do they think a cure will soon be found?

These examples, drawn from the literature reviewed in this chapter, suggest the varied and sometimes problematic beliefs individuals may hold regarding AIDS and HIV infection. The HBM suggests the importance of developing a good sense of a client's belief system in the course of counseling for behavior change. The beliefs a given client holds, as well as the theoretical model of the counselor, will then determine the specific techniques used to change those beliefs that interfere with preventive behaviors.

The effectiveness of counseling interventions will also be increased by evaluating client beliefs about preventive behaviors. If the perceived costs of using condoms, reducing the number of partners, or avoiding anal intercourse outweigh the perceived benefits, the treatment program may need to include components designed to reduce these costs. Alternately, the counselor could work to increase the perceived benefits of safe sex or safe drug use behavior. Cognitive techniques such as "eroticizing" safe sex, or skills training (e.g., effective needle cleaning or correct condom use) may affect the perceived costs and benefits of preventive practices.

Similarly, a low sense of personal efficacy will also interfere with risk behavior change. A client who feels unable to use condoms because of a lack of skills will need a different intervention from one who is concerned about communicating the need for condom use to his or her partner. In general, self-efficacy can be increased by giving clients simple tasks at which they are likely to succeed. The difficulty and complexity of tasks can be increased gardually until the person has a sense of mastery, and an ability to perform the desired preventive task. Research has shown the importance of perceiving one's peers as supportive of healthy behaviors in the initiation and maintenance of health behavior change. This may be most easily accomplished in a group format and through community-based interventions. However, individual clients can be taught how to obtain support from friends and how to recruit friends likely to be supportive of healthy behaviors. This component of the HBM, when included in an intervention program, can reinforce and maintain preventive behaviors outside of the therapy setting.

Finally, altering community norms regarding risk behavior, although difficult to achieve, may be particularly effective in enabling widespread risk reduction. The counselor's role often extends beyond the individual consulting room and into a variety of community settings such as schools, universities, and mental health and substance abuse treatment agencies. Within these communities, counselors can devise and implement broad-based HIV prevention strategies that target specific groups, and that attend to the unique needs and problems of these groups. This is not a new role for counselors, who have long been involved in multiple aspects of health and mental health prevention activities in communities across the country. Instead, it requires counselors to become increasingly active in applying preexisting community and organizational skills to the problems of HIV prevention.

References

Bandura, A. (1986). *A social foundation of thought frmtand action*. Englewood Cliffs, NJ: Prentice-Hall.

Becker, M.H. (1974). The Health Belief Model and personal health behavior. *Health Education Monographs, 2*, 324–473.

Bell, T.A., & Holmes, K.K. (1984). Age-specific risks of syphilis, gonnorhea, and hospitalized P.I.D. in sexually experienced women. *Sexually Transmitted Diseases, 11*, 291–295.

Beltangady, M. (1988). The risk of suicide in persons with AIDS. *Journal of the American Medical Association* (Letter), *260*(1), 29.

Bixler, R.E., Palacios-Jimenez, L., & Springer, E. (1987). *AIDS prevention for substance abuse treatment programs*. Narcotics and Drug Research, Inc.: 251 New Karner Road, Albany, New York.

Bolling, D.R., & Voeller, B. (1987). AIDS and heterosexual anal intercourse. *Journal of the American Medical Association* (Letter), *258*(4), 474.

Bowser, B. (1988, October). *Crack cocaine and HIV risk*. Paper presented at the Community Forum on Cocaine and AIDS, San Francisco. Sponsored by the Center for AIDS Prevention Studies, University of California, San Francisco.

Burke, D.S., Brundage, J.F., Herbold, J.R., Berner, W., Gardner, L.I., Gunzenhauser, J.D., Voskovitch, J., & Redfield, R.R. (1987). Human immunodeficiency virus infections among civilian applicants for United States military service, October 1985 to March 1986. *New England Journal of Medicine, 317*(3), 131–136.

Catania, J.A., Coates, T.J., Kegeles, S.M., Ekstrand, M., Guydish, J., & Bye, L. (1988, June). *Implications of the AIDS Risk Reduction Model for the gay community: The importance of perceived sexual enjoyment and help-seeking behaviors*. Paper presented at the Vermont Conference on Primary Prevention, Burlington, VT.

Centers for Disease Control. (1981a). Pneumocystis pneumonia—Los Angeles. *Morbidity and Mortality Weekly Reports, 30*, 250.

Centers for Disease Control. (1981b). Kaposi's sarcoma and Pneumocystis pneumonia among homosexual men—New York City and California. *Morbidity and Mortality Weekly Reports, 30*, 305–308.

Centers for Disease Control (1987). Human immunodeficiency virus infections in the United States: A review of current knowledge and plans for expansion of HIV surveillance activities. *Morbidity and Mortality Weekly Report, 36*, (Supplement S-6).

Centers for Disease Control. (1988a). World Health Organization: Global AIDS update. *CDC AIDS Weekly*, September 26.

Centers for Disease Control. (1988b). World Health Organization: Global AIDS update. *CDC AIDS Weekly*, September 12.

Centers for Disease Control. (1988c). *AIDS weekly surveillance report—United States, October 17*. Atlanta, GA: Author.

Centers for Disease Control. (1988d). Quarterly report to the Domestic Policy Council on the prevalence and rate of spread of HIV and AIDS—United States. *Morbidity and Mortality Weekly Report, 37*(6), 551–554, 559.

Centers for Disease Control. (1988e). Hudson Institute: CDC estimates criticized. *CDC AIDS Weekly*, September 5.

Centers for Disease Control. (1988f). Number of sex partners and potential risk of sexual exposure to human immunodeficiency virus. *Journal of the American Medical Association, 260*(14), 2020–2021.

Clark, H.W., & Washburn, P. (1988). Testing for human immunodeficiency virus in substance abuse treatment. *Journal of Psychoactive Drugs, 20*(2), 203–211.

Coates, T., & Greenblatt, R. (in press). Behavior change using interventions at the community level. In K. Holmes (Ed.), *Sexually transmitted diseases*. New York: McGraw-Hill.

Coates, T., Morin, S.F., & McKusick, L. (1987). Behavioral consequences of AIDS antibody testing among gay men. *Journal of the American Medical Association, 258*, 1889.

Coates, T., Stall, R., & Hoff, C. (1988). *Changes in sexual behavior of gay and bisexual men since the beginning of the AIDS epidemic*. Report to the U.S. Office of Technology Assessment. Available from first author.

Des Jarlais, D.C., & Friedman, S.R. (1987). Editorial review. HIV infection among intravenous drug users: Epidemiology and risk reduction. *AIDS, 1*, 67–76.

Des Jarlais, D.C., Friedman, S.R., Casriel, C., & Kott, A. (1987). AIDS and preventing initiation into intravenous (IV) drug use. *Psychology and Health, 1*, 179–194.

Des Jarlais, D.C., Friedman, S.R., Marmor, M., Cohen, H., Mildvan, D., Yancovitz, S., Mathur, U., El-Sadr, W., Spira, T.J., Garber, J., Beatrice, S.T., Abdul-Quader, A.S., & Sotheran, J.L. (1987). Development of AIDS, HIV seroconversion, and potential co-factors for T4 cell loss in a cohort of intravenous drug users. *AIDS, 1*, 105–111.

DiClemente, R., Zorn, J., & Temoshok, L. (1986). Adolescents and AIDS: A survey of knowledge, beliefs, and attitudes about AIDS in San Francisco. *American Journal of Public Health, 76*, 1443–1445.

Dilley, J.W., Ochitill, H.N., Perl, M., & Volberding, P.A. (1985). Findings in psychiatric consultations with patients with acquired immunodeficiency syndrome. *American Journal of Psychiatry, 142*, 82–85.

Doll, L., Darrow, W., O'Malley, P., Bodecker, T., & Jaffee, H. (1987). *Self-reported behavioral change in homosexual men in the San Francisco City Clinic Cohort*. Paper presented at the III International Conference on AIDS, Washington, DC.

Donlou, J.N., Wolcott, D.L., Gottlieb, M.S., & Landsverk, J. (1985). Psychosocial aspects of AIDS and AIDS-related complex: A pilot study. *Journal of Psychosocial Oncology, 3*, 39–55.

Ekstrand, M., & Coates, T. (1988, June). *Prevalence and change in AIDS high risk behavior among gay and bisexual men*. Paper presented at the IV International Conference on AIDS, Stockholm.

Elkind, D. (1967). Egocentrism in adolescence. *Child Development, 38*, 1024–1034.

Fox, R., Odaka, N.J., Brookmeyer, R., & Polk, B.F. (1987). Effect of HIV antibody disclosure on subsequent sexual activity in homosexual men. *AIDS, 1*, 241–246.

Friedland, G., & Klein, R. (1987). Transmission of the human immunodeficiency virus. *New England Journal of Medicine, 317*, 1125–1135.

Fullilove, M., & Fullilove, R. (1987, September). *What risk do minority adolescents face from the AIDS epidemic?* Paper presented at the NIMH Conference on Women and Health: Promoting Healthy Behaviors, Bethesda, MD.

Gibson, D.R., Wermuth, L., Lovelle-Drache, J., Ergas, B., & Sorensen, J.L. (1988, June). *Brief psychoeducational counseling to reduce AIDS risk in IV drug users and sexual partners*. Paper presented at the IV International Conference on AIDS, Stockholm.

Goldsmith, M.F. (1988). Sex tied to drugs = STD spread. *Journal of the American Medical Association, 260*(14), 2009.

Greenblatt, R., Lukehart, S., & Plummer, F. (1988). Genital ulceration as a risk factor for HIV infection. *AIDS, 2*, 42–50.

Guydish, J., Coates, T., & Ekstrand, M. (1988, June). *Changes in AIDS-related high risk behavior among heterosexual men*. Paper presented at IV International Conference on AIDS, Stockholm.

Harris, L. (1981). *American teens speak: Sex myths, TV and birth control. The Planned Parenthood poll*. New York: Planned Parenthood Federation of America.

Haverkos, H.W., & Edelman, R. (1988). The epidemiology of acquired immunodeficiency syndrome among heterosexuals. *Journal of the American Medical Association, 260*(13), 1922–1929.

Hearst, N., & Hulley, S.B. (1988). Preventing the heterosexual spread of AIDS: Are we giving our patients the best advice? *Journal of the American Medical Association, 259*(16), 2428–2432.

Hessol, N., Lifson, A., Rutherford, G.W., O'Malley, P.M., Franks, D.R., Darrow, A.R., & Jaffe, H.W. (1988, June). *Co-factors for progression of HIV infection in a cohort of homosexual and bisexual men: A decade of epidemiologic research*. Paper presented at the IV International Conference on AIDS, Stockholm.

Holland, J., & Tross, S. (1985). The psychosocial and neuropsychiatric sequelae of the acquired immunodeficiency syndrome. *Annals of Internal Medicine, 103*, 760–764.

Hubbard, R.L., Marsden, M.E., Cavanaugh, E., Rachal, J.V., & Ginzburg, H.M. (1988). Role of drug abuse treatment in limiting the spread of AIDS. *Reviews of Infectious Diseases, 10*(2), 377–384.

Jason, J., Lui, K., Ragni, M., Darrow, W., & Hessol, N. (1988, June). *Risk of developing AIDS in HIV-infected cohorts of hemophilic and homosexual men.* Poster presented at the IV International Conference on AIDS, Stockholm.

Joseph, J.G., Montgomery, S.B., Kessler, R.C., Ostrow, D.G., & Wortmen, C.B. (1988, June). *Determinants of high risk behavior and recividism in gay men.* Paper presented at the IV International Conference on AIDS, Stockholm.

Kegeles, S.M., Adler, N.E., & Irwin, C.E. (1988). Sexually active adolescents and condoms: Changes over one year in knowledge, attitudes and use. *American Journal of Public Health, 78*, 460–461.

Lemp, G.F., Hessol, N.A., Rutherford, G.W., Payne, S.F., Chen, R.T., Winkelstein, W., Wiley, J.A., Moss, A.R., Feigal, D., & Werdegar, D. (1988, June). *Projections of AIDS morbidity and mortality in San Fracisco using epidemic models.* Paper presented at the IV International Conference on AIDS, Stockholm.

Lui, K.J., Darrow, W.W., & Rutherford, W. (1988). A model-based estimate of the mean incubation period for AIDS in homosexual men. *Science, 249*(4857), 1333–1335.

Martin, J. (1987). The impact of AIDS on gay male sexual behavior patterns in New York City. *American Journal of Public Health, 77*, 578–581.

Marzuk, P.M., Tierney, H., Tardiff, K., Gross, E.M., Morgan, E.B., Hsu, M., & Mann, J. (1988). Increased risks of suicide in persons with AIDS. *Journal of the American Medical Association, 259*(9), 1333–1337.

McCusker, J., Stoddard, A.M., Mayer, K.H., Zapka, J., Morrison, C., & Saltzman, S.P. (1988). Effects of HIV antibody test knowledge on subsequent sexual behaviors in a cohort of homosexually active men. *American Journal of Public Health, 78*, 462–467.

Moss, A.R. (1987). AIDS and intravenous drug use: The real heterosexual epidemic. *British Journal of Medicine, 294*(6569), 389–390.

National Institute of Allergy and Infectious Disease (NIAID). (1980). *Sexually transmitted diseases: Summary and recommendations.* Bethesda, MD: U.S. Department of HEW, National Institute of Health.

Nichols, S. (1985). Psychosocial reactions of persons with acquired immunodeficiency syndrome. *Annals of Internal Medicine, 103*, 765–767.

Padian, N.S. (1987). Heterosexual transmission of acquired immunodeficiency syndrome: International perspectives and national projections. *Reviews of Infectious Diseases, 9*(5), 947–960.

Piot, P., Plummer, F.A., Mhalu, F.S., Lamboray, J., Chin, J., & Mann, J.M. (1988). AIDS: An international perspective. *Science, 239*, 573–579.

Plummer, F., Cameron, W., Simonsen, N., Bosire, M., Miatha, G., Kreiss, J., Waiyaki, P., Ronald, A., Ndinya-Achola, J., & Ngugi, E. (1988, June). *Co-factors in male-female transmission of HIV.* Paper presented at the IV International Conference on AIDS, Stockholm.

Puckett, S.B., & Bye, L.L. (1987). *The STOP AIDS Project: An interpersonal AIDS-prevention program.* San Francisco: The STOP AIDS Project.

Redfield, R.R., & Burke, D.S. (1988). HIV infection: The clinical picture. *Scientific American, 259*(4), 90–98.

Rosenstock, I.M., Strecher, V.J., & Becker, M.H. (1988). Social learning theory and the health belief model. *Health Education Quarterly, 15*, 175–183.

Selik, R.M., Castro, K.G., & Pappaioanou, M. (1988). Distribution of AIDS cases, by racial/ethnic group and exposure category, United States, June 1, 1981–July 4, 1988. *Morbidity and Mortality Weekly Report,* July 1988; *37* (SS No. 3), 1–10.

Simonsen, J.N., Cameron, D.W., Gakinya, M.N., Ndinya-Achola, J.O., D'Costa, L.J., Karasira, P., Cheang, M., Ronald, A.R., Piot, P., & Plummer, F.A. (1988). Human immunodeficiency virus infection among men with sexually transmitted diseases: Experience from a center in Africa. *New England Journal of Medicine, 319*(5), 274–278.

Solomon, G.F. (1985). The emerging field of psychoneuroimmunology with a special note on AIDS. *Advances, 2*, 6–19.

Solomon, G.F., & Temoshok, L. (1987). A psychoneuroimmunologic perspective on AIDS research: Questions, preliminary findings, and suggestions. *Journal of Applied Social Psychology, 17*(3), 286–308.

Sorensen, J., Gibson, D.R., Heitzmann, C., Dumontet, R., & Acampora, A. (1988, August). *AIDS prevention with drug abusers in residential treatment: Preliminary results.* Paper presented at the 96th Annual Convention of the American Psychological Association, Atlanta.

Stall, R., McKusick, L., Wiley, J., Coates, T., & Ostrow, D. (1986). Alcohol and drug use during sexual activities and compliance with safe sex guidelines for AIDS: The Behavioral Research Project. *Health Education Quarterly, 13*, 359–371.

Strunin, L., & Hingson, R. (1987). Acquired immunodeficiency syndrome and adolescents: Knowledge, beliefs, attitudes and behaviors. *Pediatrics, 79*, 825–828.

Watters, J.K. (1987). A street-based outreach model of AIDS prevention for intravenous drug users: Preliminary evaluation. *Contemporary Drug Problems, 14*(3), 411–423.

Wermuth, L., Ham, J., & Gibson, D.R. (1988, November). *AIDS prevention outreach to female partners of IV drug users.* Paper presented at the meeting of the American Public Health Association, Boston.

Winkelstein, W., Lyman, D.M., Padian, N., Grant, R., Samuel, M., Wiley, J., Anderson, R.E., Lang, W., Riggs, J., & Levy, J.A. (1987a). Sexual practices and risk of infection by the human immunodeficiency virus: The San Francisco Men's Health Study. *Journal of the American Medical Association, 257*, 321–325.

Winkelstein, W., Samuel, M., Padian, N., Wiley, J.A., Lang, W., Anderson, R.E., & Levy, J.A. (1987b). The San Francisco Men's Health Study: III. Reduction in human immunodeficiency virus transmission among homosexual/bisexual men, 1982–1986. *American Journal of Public Health*, 76(9), 685–689.

Zelnik, M., & Kantner, J.F. (1980). Sexual activity, contraceptive use and pregnancy among metropolitian area teenagers. *Family Planning Perspectives*, 12, 230–237.

Section Two

WORKING WITH SPECIFIC POPULATIONS

Section Introduction

On August 10, 1987, *Newsweek* magazine ran a lead article entitled "The Face of AIDS." The magazine's cover was plastered with pictures of men and women, young and old. The purpose of the article was to remind the magazine's readers of the people behind the Centers for Disease Control statistics. In a similar vein, this section focuses on the lives of the people imprisoned by the crisis. It covers issues that arise when a counselor works with the diverse populations of people with HIV infections.

Diversity is the key to this section. Each chapter focuses on a specific population with its own needs and a unique way of dealing with the issues of AIDS. Leading this section is a chapter by Cramer that envelops the broadest ground. In chapter 3, Cramer addresses the issues of the HIV-positive individual, spotlighting the various stages a seropositive person goes through as he or she changes from being asymptomatic to symptomatic.

The other four chapters in this section describe the plight of specific subpopulations of the larger group of HIV-infected individuals. In chapter 4 Nichols combines the issues of AIDS with the issues of being a woman in today's society. Nichols writes that "it is important for counselors to be aware that HIV-infected women are, of all persons with AIDS, perhaps the most isolated, least supported, and least cohesive group." Throughout her chapter she provides counselors with ways to address issues specific to women.

Adolescence is characterized by the need to explore and the belief in personal invulnerability. In light of what health care professionals know about the transmission of AIDS, this combination proves deadly. Slater, in chapter 5, addresses issues of adolescence, examining the thinking, beliefs, and knowledge of adolescents and how counselors can assist them in coping with their fears and confusion over AIDS. Like women with AIDS, adolescents with AIDS face many issues unique to them that also are addressed in this chapter.

Substance use and abuse still remains one of the major vectors for the HIV virus. Ted Knapp-Duncan and Grant Knapp-Duncan elaborate on the specific issues that substance users face in this time of AIDS. Chapter 6 examines not only the intravenous drug users on the street but also the "white collar" drug user. The authors pay particular attention to the difficult situation that counselors face as they work with clients contending with both failing health and a chemical dependency.

Within the groups previously mentioned (HIV seropositive, women, adolescents, and drug users), not every person with AIDS is a White, middle-class American. The HIV does not discriminate; it infects members of ethnic minority groups at a rate disproportionately greater than the minorities' representation in the general population. Jue and Kain examine issues specific to culturally sensitive counseling. Chapter 7 is both content-oriented, looking at the ways specific cultures view AIDS, and process-oriented, presenting ways in which counselors can be more attuned to the issues of particular groups not in the mainstream of society.

Although the chapters in this section describe the myriad issues important to the specific subgroups of the larger population of HIV-infected people, there is a unifying theme repeated throughout the chapters of this section. In all cases, whether working with someone symptomatic or asymptomatic, old or young, man or woman, drug abuser or recovering alcoholic, White, Black, Asian, Hispanic, or Native American, it is important that counselors remember that people with AIDS are, first and foremost, people.

Chapter 3

THE HIV-POSITIVE INDIVIDUAL

David Cramer

The AIDS epidemic has directly touched the lives of millions of people around the world. Most noticeable is the tragedy individuals afflicted with the more serious disorders experience during the advanced stages of the infection. Less visible, however, are one to two million estimated Americans who are HIV (human immunodeficiency virus) seropositive and who are asymptomatic; that is, they display no outward indications of infection. The asymptomatic individual will struggle with many of the same issues as the individual with full-blown AIDS: discrimination, death and dying, health concerns, rejection by loved ones, and, in most cases, coming out as a gay man or an IV drug user. With wider availability of anonymous testing sites, larger numbers of people are opting to receive testing in order to prepare for their future. This can result in more individuals who will seek counseling in an effort to determine if they should be tested or as an outcome of learning they are HIV-positive. This chapter will focus on the various stages of HIV-positive seroconversion in which counseling may be beneficial: pre- and posttesting for HIV antibody status, ongoing medical care, and ongoing psychotherapy with its attendant clinical issues.

Pretest Counseling

People may consider taking the HIV antibody test for various reasons. Some may believe they have been exposed to the virus due to past behaviors, which may or may not have been highly risky. For example, a fear of infection sometimes stems from a sense of punitive guilt for engaging in extramarital behavior rather than from having engaged in sexual acts thought to spread the virus. The counselor, therefore, will need to have a sound knowledge base about AIDS and how the virus is spread in order to adequately help people make decisions about testing. In addition, the differences between anonymous testing sites and confidential tests should be highlighted, so that the individual considering testing can opt for the site that offers him or her a balance between protection from discrimination and sound ongoing medical treatment. If the individual simply desires the test results for personal knowledge, then the anonymous sites offer more protection from potential discrimination. If the desire to be tested stems from strong medical concerns, and the client has a supportive ongoing medical doctor, then confidential testing as a part of a medical regimen may be preferred in order to enhance diagnosis and treatment.

The importance of sound and comprehensive counseling as a component of HIV antibody testing is based on the findings that HIV antibody testing is often followed by increased emotional distress, increased substance abuse, and vocational disruption (Coates, Morin, & McKusick, 1987a). The same authors, in a different report (Coates, Morin, & McKusick, 1987b) noted that most seropositive individuals experience anxiety, depression, insomnia, and memory problems after learning their status. In addition, suicidal thought, guilt, withdrawal, and feelings of hopelessness were commonly reported aftereffects. Therefore, it is important to keep in mind that the decision to be tested can have powerful emotional consequences. Counseling is important in providing each individual with the capabilities and resources for dealing with the behavioral and psychological results of testing.

Perry and Markowitz (1988) outlined five important components of pretest counseling: What the test actually means, confidentiality, the decision to be tested, assessing the client's strengths and weaknesses, and responding to the client's questions. The counselor who is working with clients who are considering HIV antibody testing should become familiar with each of these elements.

Clinical Measurement: What the Test Means

The two procedures most often utilized are the ELISA (enzyme-linked immunosorbent assay) and the Western Blot.

Both of these tests are conducted on a specimen of blood taken from the individual, and there is a delay of several days to 2 weeks before the lab results return. Tests that can produce more immediate results are being developed. It is important to note that these are not tests for AIDS, but tests that determine if the individual has developed antibodies to HIV, a sign that he or she has been exposed to the virus and may be infectious—capable of spreading the virus to others. The ELISA, which is the quickest and least expensive of the two measures, is usually followed by the Western Blot as a confirmatory test if the ELISA is positive. The combination of the two tests results in an accurate protocol, where the chances of a false positive result (obtaining a positive result in an individual who is not infected) are slim. However, as it may take 6 to 12 weeks or more for an individual to develop antibodies after an infection, a person who is tested during this period between infection and the development of a measurable immune response might receive a false negative (a report stating that he or she is not infected when indeed they are). Therefore, anyone who has engaged in high-risk behaviors will require repeat testing at 2-month intervals to confirm they are not infected with HIV. When an individual first tests positive, he or she is said to have seroconverted from seronegativity to seropositivity.

The pretest counseling period is the appropriate time to discuss prognosis with clients, when they are not overwhelmed with learning they are positive, or so relieved at learning they are negative that they fail to pay close attention to the counselor. The discussion of prognosis should address the fact that most people who are seropositive do not have AIDS and will not develop it in the near future. Estimates are that only 4% of the 1.5 million people thought to be HIV-positive have developed AIDS. In one study, Hessol et al. (1987) reported that 4% to 5% of HIV-positive individuals will develop AIDS each year following the initial infection. In addition, with faster intervention and new experimental drugs, an informed HIV-positive individual today will fare better medically than one who developed the infection early on in the epidemic.

Confidentiality Versus Anonymity

A discussion of confidentiality requires the counselor to be well versed about local laws pertaining to mental health privacy and discrimination related to AIDS. Present thinking on this matter is mixed, and when a counselor should consider breaching confidentiality will be discussed later in this chapter.

Counselors should be aware that medical records are confidential in much the same manner as are mental health records. This means that, with written consent from the client, outside agencies such as insurance companies can obtain these records. Thus any testing performed in a physician's office or clinic will be incorporated in the client's medical records. This can be distinguished from the anonymous testing sites, which have been established in major cities throughout the country. Anonymous sites were created to encourage individuals to seek testing and counseling without any risk that their results would become part of a medical record. When an individual contacts such a site and makes an appointment for testing, he or she is asked to give a false name or is assigned a randomly generated code number. No information is obtained that could identify the individual. The individual's privacy is thereby closely guarded.

Making the Decision

The decision to be tested is a complex process. The Centers for Disease Control (CDC) (CDC, 1987a) have proposed that people in the following categories undergo testing: men who have engaged in homosexual behavior since 1978; IV drug users; recipients of blood and blood products between 1978 and March 1985; sexual partners of any of the preceding; women from any of the preceding groups considering pregnancy; people treated for sexually transmitted diseases; patients treated for medical, psychiatric, or neurological illnesses that may be caused by HIV infection; people who have multiple sex partners; individuals who continue to engage in high-risk behaviors; and emigrants from countries where HIV infection is high. In another report, the CDC (1987b) estimated that 20%–25% of exclusively gay men are seropositive, with that figure rising as high as 68% in some locales. Sixty-five percent of people with hemophilia are thought to be seropositive, and approximately 5% of all IV drug users may be infected with HIV (in New York City it is estimated that 50%–65% of IV drug users are seropositive). The important decision to be tested can best be made after careful thought has been given to exploring the need to know. Some individuals with minimal risk (such as someone who had a blood transfusion in an area of the country not heavily affected by the epidemic) may have a strong and pressing desire to know and may be obsessed with the fear of not knowing. Another individual who has engaged in risky behavior over a long period of time may choose to adapt to a safe life style and act "as if" they are seropositive, without seeking verification. Deciding to be tested means that one must admit to oneself to having engaged in risky behavior, and one must also then deal with the fear, worry, and anxiety associated with this admission. Clients can best explore these issues in a setting where they feel safe and secure about the privacy of their counseling.

Assessing Strengths and Weaknesses

Another factor that requires discussion before testing is the individual's particular strengths and vulnerabilities that will play a role in how the person copes with the test results. The counselor should explore how the client would react to a positive or negative test result, how the client has reacted to stressful events in the past, in whom the client would confide or to whom disclose the results, and whom they would perceive to be sources of support. Does the client have an adequate support network? Does the client have negative feelings about him- or herself to the degree that a positive test result might be catastrophic? Why is the client seeking testing at this particular time? These are all valid questions for exploring the client's motivations and inner capacity for handling stress. It is important that the counselor familiarize the client with resources in the community that can provide ongoing care in the areas a client is likely to feel vulnerable.

Answering Questions

The last phase of pretest counseling involves encouraging the client to ask questions or raise any concerns that still exist. Perry and Markowitz (1988) also suggested that the client be told that the posttest session will include his or her test results and information about resources in the community. The client is then instructed to refrain from engaging in any sex or needle sharing until that session. At that time, the client can be given detailed information about how to prevent the spread of HIV, as the client will most likely be highly motivated to attend to this material once he or she knows the test results.

Posttest Counseling

The posttest counseling session can be lengthy and require well over an hour to properly help a person begin integrating the results of his or her HIV status. The session should begin with a clear statement that the client's results indicate that he or she is HIV-infected or not infected. Following this notification, it may be helpful to again outline what the test results mean and delineate the limitations of the status (i.e., it is not a test for AIDS). The immediate needs of the seropositive individual will require attention. Perry and Markowitz (1988) suggested that up to 20 minutes be given to allow the seroconverted individual time to cope with the probable initial numbness and disbelief, and any feelings of anger, fear, or despair. The counselor may need to take an active and direct stance in exploring these reactions, as even clients who had previously stated they believed they would test positive will have emotional reactions to the confirmation. It is best to begin the work of resolving these feelings immediately, because the longer they go unaddressed the more likely that maladaptive denial will be utilized to cope with the distress. A positive test result means the individual will have to struggle with life-and-death issues for the rest of his or her life, cope with uncertain and painful medical treatments, and deal with constant discrimination and rejection. Those clients who test seronegative will also require time to discuss their doubts about the test's validity and the fact that a negative result is not a protection against future infection.

The next phase of the posttest session involves a detailed discussion of how to prevent the spread of HIV. This can give the HIV-positive individual a sense of control that can counter feelings of helplessness that are often associated with this infection. This also encourages the client to act responsibly, which can result in reducing any guilt he or she may feel about past behaviors that may have spread the virus. The seronegative individual will probably be highly motivated at this point to learn the difference between risky and safer behaviors. This information should be presented clearly and directly, with the counselor making certain that the client understands the proper use of condoms, how to clean needles, and so forth. This is not a time for taking shortcuts, and the client should be engaged in a discussion of what he or she needs to alter and what problems might interfere with adopting healthy and safe behaviors. A list of resources and pamphlets that outline the above information should be given to the client.

The final consideration of posttest counseling involves assessing follow-up needs. It is important to encourage the client to maintain sound ongoing medical contact, and a solid nutritional and exercise program. The counselor should also assess the client's tendency toward self-destructive behavior. Is the seropositive individual likely to abuse alcohol or drugs as a means of coping with test results? Is the seronegative individual unable to stop from engaging in compulsive, unsafe sexual behavior? The session should be ended in a manner that encourages continuity of care and expresses confidence in the client's ability to prevent the spread of HIV.

Counseling efforts in conjunction with testing programs need to offer the HIV-positive individual immediate support and reassurance that a positive report is not a death sentence. Both pretest and posttest counseling should stress that the test is not a diagnosis of AIDS. Learning that one has a positive conversion can produce a shock-like state, and for some clients, the posttest counseling will need to help them through the resultant crisis situation. Many individuals will enter the testing protocol fully expecting a positive outcome based on their past sexual or drug usage history. For most people, however, some degree of trauma is to be expected as a result of learning such news. It is vital that those who test positive be encouraged to follow sound medical advice and a solid nutritional program and be given a list of resources they can contact in the future for financial and emotional support.

Counseling for Health Care Workers

Magallon (1987) described the necessary counseling strategies that compliment ongoing medical treatment. Her suggestions, targeted toward physicians and health care professionals, emphasize providing reassurance, education, and instruction to the HIV-positive client. Reassurance includes confirming the individual's right to privacy and confidentiality. Such guarantees can further ensure that the client will continue with regular medical treatment, which can aid in maintaining good health. Education about the virus reduces unnecessary fear and can empower the individual in making life choices. Examples of this include educating HIV-positive women about pregnancy, and educating all HIV-positive clients about safer sexual practices. Providing instruction to the client centers around prescribing behaviors that can help maintain or improve the client's physical well-being. This includes following a nutritionally sound diet that offers adequate caloric intake, engaging in a rigorous exercise program, avoiding of the use of drugs and alcohol, getting proper rest, maintaining good hygiene, and reducing stress and anxiety. All of these components are important to supporting an efficient immune system.

Counseling and Psychotherapy

The above information forms the basis for sound adjunctive counseling to testing programs and medical care. Most individuals will probably find this level of information and support sufficient in enabling them to continue to lead productive lives. However, an increasingly large percentage of HIV-positive individuals are likely to seek out ongoing counseling and psychotherapy as a means of obtaining more control over their health and making life-style decisions or because of incapacitating depression. For some, short-term treatment oriented toward introducing stress management skills, reducing anxiety and fears, and alleviating mild depression will be sufficient. However, counselors need to be prepared to provide services to individuals seeking long-term therapy, whether they were already in treatment before being tested, or whether they seek therapy as an aftermath of their test results. In addition, because the AIDS virus has affected all segments of our population, the counselor needs to be aware of ethnic and cultural factors, as well as be sensitive to factors associated with how the individual became infected. A middle-class gay man will probably have different treatment needs than the girlfriend of an IV drug user. The following guidelines are general suggestions for the counselor who is working with a client with HIV infection.

Coping With Stress

Every person has one's own individualistic manner of responding to stress. Some clients will face the stress-producing event (learning one is HIV-positive) directly and begin to make dramatic life-style changes in order to help maintain optimal functioning of their immune system. Other clients may utilize the defense mechanism of denial as a major coping strategy. Still others may experience tremendous guilt, depression, and entertain suicidal thoughts. Almost all will have to find ways of coping with enormous amounts of stress. Most likely to occur is an increase in reliance on an individual's normal defense mechanism, whether that be denial or obsessive or hysterical behavior. Common responses in addition to the above include disbelief, numbness, anger, chaos, and anxiety and fear.

Several studies (Tross, 1985; Temoshok, Mandel, Moulton, Solomon, & Zich, 1986) have reported that asymptomatic HIV-positive individuals are the most highly stressed group of people along the AIDS spectrum. This seems to be a result of feeling like one may be a walking time bomb—knowing one is not completely healthy and yet not having any serious signs of illness. People who are HIV-positive carry similar stressors to people with AIDS, yet they must also live with the uncertainty of it—when and how their infection will progress. There may exist a sense of little control over their eventual health course, and this can lead to a preoccupation with illness. Every cough, rash, or minor pain may trigger a panic reaction and fear that the infection is worsening. Other clients are relieved when, during allergy season, they develop runny noses and itchy eyes— a sign that their immune system is functioning at a healthy level. The HIV-infected individual who is on antiviral medication, such as AZT, will be reminded of this status each moment the timer goes off as a reminder to take the medication. Sleep cycles and daily patterns are interrupted at regular intervals several times a day. The often severe side effects of AZT, such as anemia, may also have a detrimental impact on psychological well-being. Those clients who receive regular T-cell counts as part of their medical regimen may struggle with anticipatory fear preceding the cell count, wondering if the number of T-cells in the system will be lower than in the previous measure. A lowered reading may cause depression as the client struggles with the fear that the immune system is weakening. The client may wonder if any life-style behaviors, nutrition patterns, or negative beliefs may have contributed to the deteriorating count. If the count has increased, there is often an overwhelming sense of relief, occasionally accompanied by a feeling that the virus is no longer in the system. This struggle points out one of the most formidable tasks with which the HIV-positive individual has to cope— how to balance a feeling of hope and positive outlook with the realistic scientific and medical facts of the infection.

Jacobson, Perry, Scavusso, and Roberts (1987) reported that asymptomatic HIV-positive individuals score two to three standard deviations above the mean on measures of psychological distress. An important function of counseling for these individuals is learning stress reduction techniques (deep muscle relaxation, autohypnosis, meditation, yoga, exercise, etc.) that can be employed on a daily basis. Coates and McKusick (1987) found that the integration of stress management techniques has led to decreased anxiety and depression, lessened high-risk sexual behavior, and increased functioning of the immune system. In addition, it is common for individuals facing a serious illness to utilize denial in coping with the fear of losing physical health. Allowing the use of denial is essential when it enables the individual to "forget" that he or she is infected with HIV, and return to a normal day-to-day routine. As such, denial should be challenged only when its use compromises good medical advice. More often than not, clients (and counselors) need to be given permission to use a little denial now and then in an effort to decrease obsessing about the virus.

Another effective component of counseling is the process of expressing emotions, also termed abreaction. Affective expression has been found effective not only in combating isolation and depression, but it may actually have an immune enhancing effect. Certainly clients who are HIV-positive can be encouraged and supported in the expression of anger and rage, both at the virus itself, as well as at social discrimination. In addition, visualization can be a supplement to treatment in much the same manner as in cancer patients (Simonton, Matthews-Simonton, & Creighton, 1980). Visualization allows the client to individualize his or her response to the virus. Some clients prefer to imagine scenes of attacking and expelling the virus. Yet other clients seem more comfortable visualizing the body accepting and pacifying the virus, as if they are turning it off. Cognitive behavioral techniques, such a thought-stopping, self-talk, and reattributions can benefit the seropositive individual by interrupting obsessive thoughts and ruminations. Other psychosocial factors, such as separation and divorce, bereavement, and relationship problems, have also been indicated as possibly affecting the functioning of the immune system (Kiecolt-Glaser & Glaser, 1988). Empowering clients by increasing the quality of their emotional and inner life can only enhance their lives and their relationships. Finally, researchers have reported on the benefits of antidepressant medication for those individuals who are immobilized by their depression (Fernandez, Levy, & Galizzi, 1988) and on the use of benzodizepine to alleviate anxiety and panic attacks (Perry & Markowitz, 1986).

Sexuality

Other challenging issues may also be brought to the therapist. A concern such as how to incorporate sexuality into one's life may actually have complex overtones involving guilt and a negative self-image. Gay men, in particular, are susceptible to experiencing feelings of self-hatred that arise out of internalized homophobia. This form of self-denigration can often go as far as believing that one has brought this infection upon oneself because of being gay. It is imperative that counselors counter these feelings by exploring what role self-hate has played in the client's upbringing and inform the client that viruses do not discriminate but attack people from all walks of life. The homophobic reaction is most often noticed as a part of the bargaining state (Kübler-Ross, 1969) where the individual agrees never to practice homosexual behaviors again if God will cure him of the virus. In this context, the goal of therapy may be to acknowledge the feelings and help the client move through this stage of grief.

Eliminating sex from one's life is another drastic method of coping with being HIV-positive. Abstinence may be a valued choice for some people, but this decision should be reached only after careful exploration of underlying motivations. Safer sexual practices can allow an individual to maintain both erotic satisfaction and sexual intimacy. Many community AIDS resource centers are now sponsoring workshops that focus on eroticizing safer sexual practices. Individuals who become infected through sexual behavior—or who have infected others—may have a lot of working through to do before they can feel good about themselves as sexual beings. This includes expressing and dealing with guilt and shame, internalized erotophobia (harboring negative feelings about sex), anger, and self-isolation from physical contact with others.

For gay men, even the adoption of safer sexual practices can be a tremendous loss to a self-image that was previously highly sexualized. Most gay men have had to strive to overcome indoctrination early in life that homosexuality is an abnormal perversion. One important means of countering these negative messages has been the open and free expression and exploration of sexuality, often in the form of multiple partners and various sexual acts that unfortunately can pass the virus from one person to another. The loss of this important source of self-affirmation and countering homophobic messages means that gay men have to rely more on other methods of boosting self-esteem (work, school, peers, spirituality). The giving up of past sexual behaviors results in a void that has to be filled in alternative ways by other facets of daily life. In addition, the gay man who has not yet developed a positive self-identity may experience difficulty proceeding with the coming-out process and forming an integrated view of himself. Again, the counselor can challenge this retardation as a sign of internalized homophobia. Heterosexual HIV-infected individuals will also struggle with how to maintain a healthy, rewarding, and safe sexual relationship with their partners. The counselor should actively inquire as to how the client's sexual behaviors are affected by the knowledge of HIV infection, because feelings of anger, shame, and fear may initially surface in the ways the client changes his or her sexual activity. These changes may take place on a broad spectrum, ranging from unnecessary withdrawal and isolation to uncontrollable and unsafe sexual acting-out. The counselor should avoid moralizing or scolding a client for engaging in unsafe behavior and should work to help the client deal with his or her sexuality as an inherently positive component of life. Instructing clients on safer sex and encouraging integration of these practices into relationships can provide clients with an element of control in their life, giving them behavioral choices they can practice and master, while enabling them responsibly to stop the spread of the virus and continue their personal growth.

Confidentiality and Legal Concerns

Another difficult issue in counseling and psychotherapy involves how to inform others and who should be informed of the client's antibody status. Although it is preferable that the individual not be alone in his or her efforts to adapt to living with the virus, it is also imperative to be cautious about who is told given society's tendency to react negatively to AIDS-related issues. Telling too many people can result in problems such as loss of job and income, home, and friends. Therefore, landlords, employers, co-workers, everyday acquaintances, and young children probably should not be informed. Health care workers involved in treating the client such as physicians, nurses, dentists, and paramedics will need to be told in order to ensure effective medical treatment. The client may also want to discuss with his or her health care workers how this information will be recorded in medical or psychological records and when this information might be released to other agencies such as insurance companies or the military. The medical and mental health records will need to reflect an accurate course of treatment while counselors and health care workers remain sensitive to a client's need for protection.

Each individual will need to make responsible and careful decisions about how to inform significant others, partners and spouses, close friends, and family members. The chances of a particular person providing support or rejecting the client need to be carefully weighed. Role-playing difficult disclosure situations can help the client make decisions about the best way to inform those necessary to tell and decide whom not to tell. Although it seems responsible for the client to inform lovers, a spouse or partner, some will choose not to do so. This places the counselor in a difficult situation if the couple is not practicing safer sex. This disregard for spreading the virus may be a sign of other serious problems in the relationship between the HIV-positive individual and his or her partner, and the counselors should explore how anger is expressed in the relationship and what sources of dissatisfaction exist. The issue of confidentiality is also pertinent at this point. Counselors must struggle with their own discomfort and anger at the client who knowingly continues to engage in behavior that will possibly spread the virus. It is important that the counselor address this issue in a direct yet empathetic and nonpunitive manner that encourages the client to resolve his or her rage in a more responsible way. Several authors (Girard, Keese, Traver, & Cooksey, 1988; Kain, 1988) have noted that under these circumstances the counselor does not seem to have a duty to warn other parties. Melton (1988) pointed out that no legal or judicial cases have provided guidance on how therapists should respond to this situation. It is possible that breaking confidentiality to warn others may result in more harm than good by damaging the therapeutic relationship. If an HIV-positive client continues to engage in unsafe sexual practices, the counselor may first want to consult with the ethics committee of his or her professional organization before breaking confidentiality. Local laws may provide public health officials with the power to act to prevent an individual from spreading HIV infection, so that if the counselor feels he or she needs to act to halt the client's behavior, reporting to these authorities may be the best recourse. In addition, if custody or visitation privileges are involved, the client would probably benefit from legal consultation before informing former partners of the HIV status.

Other legal issues that the counselor may want to address with his or her client include discussing the need for the client to have a will and authorizing a designated individual to have power of attorney. The latter procedure is particularly important for gay men or unmarried couples. This can provide some peace of mind and protect the client should his or her medical state worsen. Many gay couples without such protection have experienced family members taking over all rights to making medical decisions. In many cases, the wishes of the ill individual and the gay partner have been rejected by homophobic family members. The power of attorney can legally invest a partner of a trusted friend with the authority to make certain medical and legal decisions, such as which medical interventions can be used and what rights of visitation apply, so that the patient's wishes are preserved. Although taking such legal steps is in the best interest of the client, the counselor needs to take cues from the client about when he or she is ready to make such decisions. In addition, these measures should be approached in a proactive, affirming manner designed to provide clients with more control over their lives, and not as a step toward preparing for immediate death. These are actions that would benefit all people (not only the HIV-infected) in preparing for eventual death.

Countertransference

The counselor's own attitude and feelings toward HIV-positive clients will be of primary importance in allowing the establishment of a safe a trusting therapeutic relationship.

Counselors need to be aware that little is known about the course of AIDS, and that a large percentage of antibody-positive individuals have lived many years with no symptomatology. In addition, others have developed mild symptoms only to see them disappear with medical treatment.

This points to the importance of instilling in the client a positive, life-enhancing outlook. In fact, Faltz and Madover (1987) suggested that many individuals who previously had led lives encumbered by severe drug and alcohol use and shallow relationships have greatly enhanced the quality of their day-to-day endeavors since learning they were HIV-positive. Although AIDS can be devastating, we do not know it to be a sure death sentence. The importance of positive thinking and an affirmative life style have been shown to be effective adjuncts in treating life-threatening chronic illnesses (Seigal, 1986). Therefore, it is important for the counselor to pay attention to his or her own feelings regarding countertransference, which may be more subtle and hidden when working with an asymptomatic individual as compared to someone with full-blown AIDS. The counselor will probably have to deal with his or her own concerns about fear, uncertainty, anxiety, anger, homosexuality, drugs, and death. Rosse (1985) found that 73% of inpatient psychiatric staff harbored fears of contagion through casual contact even thought medical science has consistently shown that transmission of the virus is limited to blood-to-blood or semen-to-blood contact.

Faltz and Madover (1987) discussed two other powerful countertransference issues: the need for professional omnipotence and overidentification with the client. The former concern has to do with the therapist's own helplessness to sometimes effectively enable people to change behaviors or to ultimately alter the course of the HIV infection. For unknown reasons, some individuals who seem to have adopted healthy behaviors and attitudes still advance to a more serious level of the infection. It can be extremely difficult for both the client and the caring counselor to accept a transition from being HIV-positive to being diagnosed with AIDS. The resultant crisis will demand an immediate response to cope with the advance of the infection to this level. The transition from HIV-positive status to AIDS can be a frustrating and drawn-out expensive experience that involves numerous tests, procedures, and doctors. Haney (1988) noted that after going through such an ordeal, most clients expect to be prepared for the AIDS diagnosis. What often occurs, however, is another severe crisis during which psychological support is crucially needed to prevent fear and anger from turning into self-destructive behavior. Overidentification with the client can occur particularly when the counselor shares common concerns in his or her own life, such as "Am I infected with the virus?" Problems for counselors in this situation include pushing the client toward changes too fast or letting their own values dominate clinical decisions. Counselors who are at risk for HIV infections need to take care of their own concerns, independently of their relationships with their clients.

Another difficult situation for the counselor involves having to confront an "ill" individual when the individual is engaging in behaviors that are not therapeutic. Some counselors may be reluctant to bring up difficult issues when working with a client who is already coping with multiple stressors. However, the counselor's position with the client may be vital in that he or she may be the only person in the client's life willing to bring up unpleasant topics such as drug and alcohol use and unsafe sexual behavior. Discussing these behaviors provides an opportunity to deepen the therapeutic relationship and enables the client to learn more about his or her manner of relating to others. In addition, counselors need to remain cognizant of their dual responsibility to the client and to society at large. Bohm (1987) pointed out that educated HIV-positive individuals who continue unsafe sexual behavior are engaging in denial and expressing their anger. Therapy in this case should not avoid the issues but focus on the underlying motivations behind unsafe activities. This includes exploring why such clients have chosen to expose themselves and others to the virus, and what is occurring in their life that is causing them to engage in repeated attempts to risk their own or others' lives. The counselor should ask the clients about sexual or drug-related behavior, even if the clients do not volunteer this information. This reinforces that the counselor places a high priority on stopping the spread of the virus.

Every individual has his or her own characteristic manner of reponding to stress. Some will cope with pain and stress through increased risky behaviors, such as compulsive sexual activity or abusing drugs and alcohol. Others may withdraw and isolate themselves or engage in increased hypochondriacal complaints. The counselor will need to assess the client's ability to cope with stress by evaluating past relationships, education and career achievements, level of self-esteem and identity formation, previous coping skills, and the degree of support from caring others. The degree of development of the client's own psychological characteristics will play a major role in determining how the individual tolerates the uncertainty of being HIV-positive. Faltz and Madover (1987) emphasized that the crisis brought on by learning one is HIV-positive may prove to be the opportunity to enhance one's life tremendously. The counselor, while adopting an optimistic outlook, should avoid minimizing or denying the real fears and anxieties of the seropositive individual.

Special Considerations

Other concerns will often need to be addressed in counseling to fully provide a broad-spectrum intervention for the client. These issues include: the needs of significant others, specific concerns for women, suicide, central nervous system (CNS) impairment, and group therapy. The counselor may often be involved not only with working with the antibody client, but also his or her spouse or partner and family members. The client's significant others, who are most often the primary caregivers, will also experience grief and an adaptation period (Fuller, Geis, & Rush, 1988; Greif & Porembski, 1988). Many communities also offer support groups for the loved ones of those infected by the virus. These groups serve not only to counter isolation but also to dispel blame and guilt and provide information. In addition, some groups have formed for those who are survivors of losing a loved one to AIDS. Many HIV-positive clients indeed already have lost their partner or numerous friends. Grieving is a natural healing process and as such, can be fostered in the therapeutic alliance with a trusted counselor.

Women who test positive for the AIDS antibody should be counseled about the chronicity of the infection and the chances of passing the virus on to offspring during pregnancy or at the time of delivery. Kapila and Kloser (1988) cited a 50% chance that the infant of an HIV-positive woman would also harbor the virus. Additionally, women who are considering artificial insemination by a donor should take precautions to screen donors for HIV.

The HIV-positive individual faces many difficult and seemingly insurmountable problems. People with this infection are among the highest at risk to attempt taking their own lives, and each counselor should be proactive in assessing the possibility of such action by the client (Flavin & Francis, 1987). Suicidal ideation is likely to occur both at the moment of diagnosis, when the crisis seems overwhelming to the client, as well as at any time following the news of seroconversion. Repeated rejection by friends and loved ones, death of loved ones, societal oppression, discrimination, and a worsening physical state can all trigger feelings of hopelessness and a desire to have some control over how one dies. In addition, some individuals contemplate suicide because of the shame they feel about developing AIDS and being exposed as either IV drug users or gay. Suicidal tendencies may also surface in less obvious, yet seriously self-destructive behaviors such as drug and alcohol abuse, continued exposure to repeated infection by the virus, or other forms of life-risking behaviors as a means of coping with stress.

It has been well established that the AIDS virus crosses the blood-brain barrier and enters the central nervous system. Many HIV-infected individuals may begin to show early signs of CNS involvement, including mild cognitive impairment, forgetfulness, decreased concentration, and short-term memory loss. The counselor may have difficulty discerning if these symptoms are caused by anxiety and depression or by advancing illness. It is important to note that in some individuals, cognitive impairment and AIDS dementia are the first indications of deterioration (Wolcott, 1986; Christopher, 1988). If the symptoms persist and seem nonremedial to counseling, then a neurological referral is appropriate to determine the severity and course of the cognitive impairment.

Lastly, an important component of treating the HIV-infected individual involves referring the client to a supportive group experience. A variety of group formats have been used and shown effective in countering isolation, providing education, and decreasing risky behavior. If possible, it is more effective to offer separate groups for individuals who are affected differently by the virus. Spector and Conklin (1987) advised that asymptomatic HIV-positive people not be mixed with people with AIDS because the presence of individuals with an advanced illness often intensifies the fears of others, motivating them to drop out of the group early. Because significant others have their own special concerns, often groups are organized just for their needs (Klein & Fletcher, 1987). In addition, gay men, women, and IV drug users typically have different life styles and issues to resolve, and it is common to offer separate group experiences for each. Galea, Lewis, and Baker (1988) reported that a discussion group format proved helpful in treating long-term substance abusers. They found that the group showed increased health concerns in a population where health is usually not considered important. Those who remained in the group also had a greater rate of staying in treatment, because dropping out of the group could mean a return to behavior that might lead to infection. Other authors (Lauers-Listhaus & Watterson, 1988; Posey, 1988) also reported that the psychoeducational group experience is effective in dealing with reducing behavior that may pass the virus on to others as well as providing a powerful format for confronting other forms of self-destructive behavior (Price, Omizo, & Hammett, 1986). The group experience may be the only haven a client or significant other has that provides acceptance, safety, and reassurance while dispelling the blame and guilt often associated with AIDS.

Conclusion

The effort to provide counseling and psychotherapy to the HIV-positive client calls upon our most human traits and can challenge our own feelings about our sexuality and mortality. The counselor must convey a hopeful, positive, and caring attitude that in itself can be healing without minimizing the real and painful struggles the client has to endure. Life is a fragile existence that can be lost at any moment. For the HIV-positive client, the struggle centers around how to live life deeply and with meaning in the here-and-now while preparing for an uncertain future. As therapists, it is our responsibility to prevent this virus from destroying self-respect.

References

Bohm, E. (1987). AIDS: Effects on psychotherapy in New York City. *Journal of Psychosocial Nursing, 25,* 26–31.

Centers for Disease Control. (1987a). Public health service guidelines for counseling and antibody testing to prevent HIV infection and AIDS. *Morbidity and Mortality Weekly Report, 36,* 509–515.

Centers for Disease Control. (1987b). Human immunodeficiency virus infection in the United States. *Morbidity and Mortality Weekly Report, 36*, 802–804.

Christopher, J. (1988). Assault on the brain. *Psychology Today, 22*, 38–39, 42–44.

Coates, T., & McKusick, L. (1987). *The efficacy of stress management in reducing high risk behavior and improving immune function in HIV antibody positive men.* Paper presented to the III International Conference on AIDS, Washington, DC.

Coates, T., Morin, S., & McKusick, L. (1987a). Behavioral consequences of AIDS antibody testing among gay men. *Journal of the American Medical Association, 258*, 1889.

Coates, T., Morin, S., & McKusick, L. (1987b). *Consequences of AIDS antibody testing among gay men: The AIDS Behavioral Research Project.* Paper presented to the III International Conference on AIDS, Washington, DC.

Faltz, B., & Madover, S. (1987). Treatment of substance abuse in patients with HIV infection. *Advances in Alcohol and Substance Abuse, 6*, 23–32.

Fernandez, F., Levy, J., & Galizzi, H. (1988). Response of HIV-related depression to psychostimulants: Case reports. *Hospital and Community Psychiatry, 39*, 628–631.

Flavin, D., & Francis, R. (1987). Risk-taking behavior, substance abuse disorders, and the acquired immune deficiency syndrome. *Advances in Alcohol and Substance Abuse, 6*, 23–32.

Fuller, R., Geis, S., & Rush, J. (1988). Lovers of AIDS victims: A minority group experience. *Death Studies, 12*, 1–7.

Galea, R., Lewis, B., & Baker, L. (1988). Voluntary testing for HIV antibodies among clients in long-term substance abuse treatment. *Social Work, 33*, 265–268.

Girard, J., Keese, R., Traver, L., & Cooksey, D. (1988). Psychotherapist responsibility in notifying individuals at risk for exposure to HIV. *Journal of Sex Research, 25*, 1–27.

Greif, G., & Porembski, E. (1988). Implications for therapy with significant others of persons with AIDS. *Journal of Gay and Lesbian Psychotherapy, 1*, 79–86.

Haney, P. (1988). Providing empowerment to the person with AIDS. *Social Work, 33*, 251–253.

Hessol, N., Rutherford, G., O'Malley, P., Doll, L., Darrow, W., & Jaffe, H. (1987). *The natural history of human immunodeficiency virus infection in a cohort study of homosexual and bisexual men: A 7-year prospective study.* Paper presented to the III International Conference on AIDS, Washington, DC.

Jacobson, P., Perry, S., Scavusso, D., & Roberts, R. (1987). *Psychological reactions of individuals at risk for AIDS during an experimental drug trial.* Paper presented at to the III International Conference on AIDS, Washington, DC.

Kain, C. (1988). To breach or not to breach: Is that the question? A response to Gray & Harding. *Journal of Counseling and Development, 66*, 224–225.

Kapila, R., & Kloser, P. (1988). Women and AIDS: An overview. *Medical Aspects of Human Sexuality, 22*, 92–103.

Kiecolt-Glaser, J., & Glaser, R. (1988). Psychological influences on immunity: Implications for AIDS. *American Psychologist, 43*, 892–898.

Klein, S., & Fletcher, W. (1987). *The importance of supportive interventions for caregiving family/friends during the AIDS crisis.* Paper presented to the III International Conference on AIDS, Washington, DC.

Kübler-Ross, E. (1969). *On death and dying.* New York: Macmillan.

Lauers-Listhaus, B., & Watterson, J. (1988). A psychoeducational group for HIV-positive patients on a psychiatric service. *Hospital and Community Psychiatry, 39*, 776–777.

Magallon, D. (1987). Counseling patients with HIV infections. *Medical Aspects of Human Sexuality, 21*, 129–147.

Melton, G. (1988). Ethical and legal issues in AIDS related practice. *American Psychologist, 43*, 941–947.

Perry, S., & Markowitz, J. (1988). Psychiatric interventions for AIDS-spectrum disorders. *Hospital and Community Psychiatry, 39*, 731–739.

Posey, C. (1988). Confidentiality in an AIDS support group. *Journal of Counseling and Development, 65*, 226–227.

Price, R., Omizo, M., & Hammett, V. (1986). Counseling clients with AIDS. *Journal of Counseling and Development, 65*, 96–97.

Rosse, R.B. (1985). Reactions of psychiatric staff to an AIDS patient (Letter). *American Journal of Psychiatry, 142*, 523.

Seigal, B. (1986). *Love, medicine, and miracles.* New York: Harper & Row.

Simonton, O.C., Matthews-Simonton, S., & Creighton, J. (1980). *Getting well again.* New York: Bantam Books.

Spector, I., & Conklin, R. (1987). AIDS group psychotherapy. *International Journal of Group Psychotherapy, 37*, 433–439.

Temoshok, L., Mandel, J., Moulton, J., Solomon, G., & Zich, J. (1986). *A longitudinal psychosocial study of AIDS and ARC in San Francisco: Preliminary results.* Paper presented at the annual meeting of the American Psychiatric Association, Washington, DC.

Tross, S. (1985). The psychological impact of AIDS: Research findings. *Outlook* (Newsletter of the Department of Psychiatry, New York Hospital, Cornell Medical Center), Spring/Summer, p. 8.

Wolcott, D. (1986). Psychosocial aspects of acquired immune deficiency syndrome and the primary care physician. *Annals of Allergy, 57*, 98–102.

Chapter 4

THE FORGOTTEN SEVEN PERCENT: WOMEN AND AIDS

Margaret Nichols

Introduction: Five Case Vignettes

Sylvia, a Black woman, divorced her first husband, a drug addict, 6 years ago and remarried a non-drug using man shortly thereafter. Two years ago she began to exhibit vague symptoms that were incorrectly diagnosed as psychosomatic. It did not occur to either her or her physician that she might be HIV-infected, so she was psychiatrically hospitalized with a diagnosis of bulimia, due to her frequent vomiting. Last spring Sylvia's ex-husband called her to inform her of his HIV seropositive status. She died within a month of learning that her symptoms were HIV-related, rather than psychiatric. Her grief-stricken second husband, himself now seropositive, apparently infected by Sylvia, now cares for his two children from a previous marriage as well as two children from Sylvia's first marriage.

Susan, a 29-year-old White working class woman, also suffered symptoms that were misdiagnosed for a year. In her third month of pregnancy, Susan mentioned to her doctor that she had had several different sexual partners since adolescence. On the basis of this clue, her doctor finally referred her for HIV antibody testing, and Susan received an ARC diagnosis when her test results were positive. Only at this point did her steady male sexual partner of 4 years, the father of her child, admit his past homosexual behavior. He told Susan that he had been afraid to tell her because he was afraid she would leave him.

He also said that he never considered himself to be at risk for AIDS because "AIDS happens to homosexuals, not bisexuals." Bobby, Susan's boyfriend, subsequently was diagnosed with ARC himself. Susan was told, in her fourth month of pregnancy, that if she carried her baby to term, both she and the baby would probably die. Frantic, she left on her own to seek an abortion, but was unable to find a clinic that would agree to perform the more complicated second trimester procedure on an HIV-infected woman. In her fifth month, on the same day she finally found a clinic that would perform the abortion, Susan's baby moved inside her for the first time and she was unable to go through with the abortion. Susan's daughter was born in August and was healthy when Susan was first interviewed by a counselor. Susan, however, had contracted toxoplasmosis in September. When Susan recovered from this opportunistic infection, she said that, on her good days, she thought about having a second baby. She believed, incorrectly, that if her daughter remained healthy, a second child would also be healthy. On the other hand, Susan also sensed subconsciously that if her baby became ill, she would feel a desperate need to try to replace her sick baby with a healthy one. For Susan, being a mother was life-affirming and helped her maintain a hopeful attitude toward her own illness, an attitude that ironically was psychologically adaptive in many ways though it might have led to another dangerous pregnancy. Eventually, all three—Susan, Bobby, and the baby—developed full-blown AIDS.

Clarissa is 23, a Puerto Rican woman who lived in Jersey City, New Jersey, one of the top 10 cities in terms of the number of AIDS cases. Like Sylvia, her first husband was an addict. Clarissa learned she was seropositive when she was routinely tested during pregnancy. Her deep religiosity, among other things, prevented her from aborting this pregnancy, and her first child was born with AIDS. Soon after this birth, her first husband died of AIDS. When Clarissa's little boy was a year old, she met another man who, from Clarissa's point of view, fell in love with her and moved in to live with her and support her despite her seropositive status. Clarissa's new partner asked to have a second child—he wanted her to have his baby—and Clarissa complied. She never considered not complying, in fact, and left her fate, in her view, in the hands of God. When Clarissa was 7 months pregnant, her little boy died.

Nancy, a 28-year-old White nurse practitioner, came from an upper-middle class professional background. One day all the nurses who worked in her office, concerned about past needle-sticks, decided to go as a group to take the HIV antibody test. Two weeks later Nancy was dumbstruck to learn that she tested positive. For a long time she racked her brain to try to imagine how she had been exposed to HIV. She began to call all her past boyfriends and, finally, when she contacted a man she had been involved with 7 years earlier, she learned that, unbeknownst to her, he had been an IV drug user and that he too was antibody positive. Soon after, Nancy began to develop the symptoms of ARC. She first reacted by withdrawing and isolating herself, feeling alienated from her peers who, in fact, did not know how to handle this situation. Nancy then joined a peer support group for people with AIDS and ARC. She was the only woman in the group—the rest were gay men or male IV drug users–but Nancy didn't care. These men became her new peer support group, and eventually Nancy turned her depression and isolation into action: she did AIDS volunteer work and participated in AIDS-related political activities.

Cindy, 20, grew up in a poor White family where she was physically and sexually abused. By the age of 12 she was a runaway, sleeping in abandoned cars. Her husband is an addict who was diagnosed with AIDS when their baby was 5 months old. Cindy, Richard, and the baby have an income of $136 per month from local welfare because Richard's Social Security disability benefit was denied when his clinic doctor filled out the paperwork incorrectly. Cindy and the baby are healthy, but Cindy didn't want Richard to use condoms in their sexual relationship even after his diagnosis. During group counseling, Cindy verbalized her fantasy that, if she contracted AIDS, her abusive and neglectful family might "come around" and care for her in a way they had never loved her as a child. The group persuaded her to give up this fantasy and she began to have safer sex with Richard.

Epidemiology of AIDS in Women

Although women compose only 7% of all reported AIDS patients in the United States, they are an important potential source for heterosexual HIV transmission as well as the source of transmission to infants. In New York City in late 1987, for example, one in 61 infants was born with the antibodies to the AIDS virus (Brooks-Gunn, Boyer, & Hine, 1988). Moreover, recent trends indicate increases in sexually transmitted cases in U.S.-born women, suggesting an increase in the heterosexual transmission of the AIDS virus to women (Hardy & Guinan, 1987).

To some extent, the relatively low overall percentage of female AIDS cases in the United States (compared to, for example, the 50% rate in parts of Africa) is misleading because it reflects primarily the fact that AIDS in this country was first diagnosed among gay men. Here, areas in which AIDS is found among intravenous drug users tend to have a higher percentage of women, reflecting not only the incidence of AIDS among female drug users but also heterosexual transmission from male addicts to their partners. New Jersey, where 17% of AIDS cases are women, has the highest percentage of female AIDS cases; New York, another state with many intravenous drug user cases (IVDUs) has 11% female AIDS patients.

The 7% overall figure for women has remained stable since 1982. If one analyzes risk factors for heterosexual men and women, (see Table 1), it is clear that intravenous drug use is the primary transmission mode (52%) for women, just as it is for men (68%). The most noteworthy differences in risk factors between men and women are that a higher percentage of women contracted AIDS through heterosexual sexual contact than did men (21% versus 1%). In absolute numbers, female sexual transmission cases outnumber male cases by a ratio of five to one.

TABLE 1

Heterosexual Men and Women With AIDS by Sex and Transmission Category 1981–1986

Risk Group	Men	Women	M-F Ratio
IVDU	68%	52%	4:1
Heterosexual contact	1%	21%	0.2:1
Endemic area	8%	6%	4:1
Hemophiliac	4%	<1%	33:1
Transfusions	6%	10%	2:1
Undetermined	12%	11%	3:1
Total Cases	5,358	729	3:1

Note: From "Epidemiology of AIDS in Women in the United States, 1981 through 1986" by M.E. Guinan and A.M. Hardy, 1987, *Journal of the American Medical Association, 257,* p. 2040. Copyright 1987 by the AMA. Adapted by permission.

It is difficult to interpret these data accurately, and indeed their interpretation remains one of the unanswered questions about AIDS transmission in this country. One theory that has been advanced to explain the disparate rates of U.S. female versus male heterosexual sexual transmission holds that it is merely an artifact of the stage of the epidemic we happen to be in at this time. That is, we know that AIDS first appeared in this country in mass numbers among gay men—who primarily transmit to other men—and via shared needles among intravenous drug users, 75% to 80% of whom are men. Thus it is logical that the first AIDS victims would overwhelmingly be men, but it does not mean that at some later stage in the epidemic male to female ratios could not be equal. Another theory holds that female-to-male vaginal intercourse may be a much less efficient mode of transmission than is male-to-female transmission. If this is true, there may never be as many female AIDS cases as there are male, but there will always be more women who acquire AIDS through sexual transmission than heterosexual men.

Table 2 shows risk factors of the male partners who presumably infected women who contracted AIDS through heterosexual activity. As one would expect, the majority of these male partners were intravenous drug users. A much smaller percentage were bisexual men. A comparatively large percentage—16%—reported basically unknown risks, and this is significant because, as will be discussed a bit later, women often tend not to know how they have been infected.

If one analyzes the epidemiological data on women with AIDS in order to predict future trends, one sees that, over time, higher percentages of women have become infected with AIDS via a sexual route versus other risk factors, with no correspond-

TABLE 2

AIDS in Women: Heterosexual Transmission
C.D.C. Statistics
Risk Factors for Heterosexual Contacts

Intravenous drug user	67%
Bisexual men	16%
Hemophiliac men	1%
Other/unreported risks	16%

Note: From "Epidemiology of AIDS in Women in the United States, 1981 through 1986" by M.E. Guinan and A.M. Hardy, 1987, *Journal of the American Medical Association, 257,* p. 2041. Copyright 1987 by the AMA. Adapted by permission.

ing increase in heterosexual transmission in men (see Table 3). Moreover, there is a 10-month doubling time for the mostly female heterosexual transmitted cases as opposed to a 14-month doubling time for gay male and intravenous drug user cases (Hardy & Guinan, 1987). In other words, in the future, heterosexual women who contract AIDS sexually will be a rapidly multiplying risk group that could theoretically grow to compose as many AIDS cases as are now seen among gay men and drug users. Of course, if this happens, there will be a correspondingly rapid rise in the number of infants born infected—a phenomenon already occurring in New York City.

When one looks at other characteristics of women with AIDS, one sees that AIDS is not spread evenly among racial or social classes, as it is more or less among gay men. Overall, both male and female heterosexuals with AIDS in the United States tend to be people of color—half Black and about one quarter Hispanic. As one would expect, children with AIDS are young: AIDS affects women in their childbearing years, with one third of women with AIDS being 29 years old or younger and another 45% between the ages of 30 and 39 (Guinan & Hardy, 1987).

These data reflect the fact that there are currently in the United States two major, and only somewhat overlapping, AIDS epidemics. One is among homosexually active men who are infecting mostly each other (although not exclusively) and whose behavior has changed so drastically that the rate of newly infected people in this group is probably very small. The second epidemic is among poor, minority people in urban centers where intravenous drug use and shared needle use is common. This

TABLE 3

Significant Trends in AIDS in Women
1982–1987
(p < 0.05)

	1982	1986
Increase in U.S.-born heterosexual contacts	14.0%	26.0%
Increase in mean age	30 yrs.	35.6 yrs.
Decrease in female IVDUs	59.0%	48.0%
Decrease in foreign-born heterosexual women	18.0%	5.0%

Note: From "Epidemiology of AIDS in Women in the United States, 1981 through 1986" by M.E. Guinan and A.M. Hardy, 1987, *Journal of the American Medical Association, 257*, p. 2040. Copyright 1987 by the AMA. Adapted by permission.

epidemic started with mostly male and some female drug users, and the female drug users' children, but is spreading to include women who are not drug users but who have been the sexual partners of drug users, and their children. Depending upon factors such as the ease of female-to-male transmission and rates of female partner change, this "second epidemic" could eventually outstrip and dwarf the first. If unchecked it could become a disease of poor minority heterosexuals and their children who live in urban centers. This is the most likely spread to the so-called "general population." Whether this epidemiological spread will continue into the White heterosexual middle class will depend upon factors such as rates of intravenous drug use among the middle class, and rates of sexual contacts across racial barriers and across social classes.

Another source of spread to White middle-class women is through the activity of functionally bisexual men, both men who label themselves bisexual (a very small percentage of all men), men who identify as heterosexuals but who have clandestine homosexual activity, and men who identify themselves as gay but have some continuing heterosexual activity. The approximately 3% of women with AIDS who contracted AIDS through bisexual men are a harbinger of this trend, which, through tertiary female-to-male sexual spread, could introduce a new type of risk group: White middle-class heterosexuals whose only source of infection is sexual contact with other White non-drug using heterosexuals. It is impossible to predict the rate or likelihood of substantial spread in this way presently because there are too many unknown, unmeasured variables that could affect this transmission, including the true rate of bisexual activity in the United States. Part of the difficulty in describing or predicting the course of the AIDS epidemic among women (and thus among children and non-intravenous drug using heterosexuals) lies in the fact that there are so few cohort studies of women such as the ones in progress studying AIDS among gay men. In the absence of such studies, counselors must piece together a picture of women and AIDS from bits of data gathered in high incidence areas. Among the most relevant statistics are the following:

- In New York City AIDS is the leading cause of death for all women between 25–34 years of age (Kristal, 1986);
- A sample of women with AIDS at Montefiore Hospital in New York showed that 35 women had a total of 52

dependent children. This underscores the fact that women with AIDS don't simply bear infected children, but they also already have other children. In fact, the problem of "AIDS orphans" is a much bigger problem in numbers than that of pediatric AIDS (Friedland, 1985).

- Women who are HIV-infected stand a 35% to 50% chance of bearing an infected infant (Peckham, Sentuvia, & Ades, 1987). Moreover, most pregnant seropositive women choose not to terminate their pregnancies, even when informed of the risk. A study in New York reported that of 80 pregnant seropositive women only one chose to abort. These figures reflect the tremendous role that motherhood plays in the lives of women who do not have access to other social roles or to other sources of self-esteem, pleasure, and life gratification. Moreover, to many poor women whose lives are already full of risk, even the 50–50 odds of having a healthy baby represent a comparatively acceptable risk. Coupled with these factors are variables such as religious beliefs about abortion and mistrust of doctors and health authorities who convey risk information.

- A study done at Downstate Medical Center in New York (Landesman, Minkoff, Holman, McCalia, & Sijin, 1987) that matched both subjects' and interviewers' judgments about a woman's serostatus with actual serostatus as determined by blood samples showed that the interviewers were not able to classify 42% of the at-risk women properly and that two thirds of the women themselves were unaware of a positive antibody status. Only intravenous drug-using women were both aware of their own risk and seemed obviously at risk to the trained interviewers. In other words, women who became HIV-infected through sexual transmission were usually unaware that they were at risk. This is probably because, in general, the pattern of sexual transmission to women is different from that to gay men. Both Padian et al. (1987) and Cohen, Hauer, Poole, and Wofsy (1987) found that, unlike among gay men, having multiple sexual partners is not the highest risk factor for women. Most women who have contracted AIDS sexually and who have not had multiple partners have become infected by multiple exposures over time to a new infected man who was either unaware himself of his risk status or was deceiving his female partner.

Thus, for women, so-called "promiscuity" does not at this time seem to be related to infection. Unfortunately, this is not widely known, and women who are in what they consider to be monogamous, stable relationships are probably lulled into a false sense of security by the media emphasis upon multiple partners as a risk factor for AIDS.

• Although anal sex is probably a more efficient route of transmission than vaginal sex (Padian et al., 1987), it is clear that vaginal sex is sufficient. It also seems, from the few data collected, that it takes, on the average, a rather large number of exposures for women to become infected through vaginal intercourse. Moreover, it seems clear that condom use does provide protection (Fischl, Dickinson, Scott, Klimas, Fletcher, & Parks, 1987). However, because the precise route of transmission to women is unknown—particularly whether transmission takes place through the vagina, cervix, or uterine lining—other mechanisms of prevention for women cannot be confidently recommended. This presents great difficulties to women because they must persuade their male partners to use condoms instead of having a method (e.g., diaphragm with spermicidal jelly, cervical sponge) that they can use themselves.

Counseling Women About AIDS: Prevention

In the absence of comprehensive data, counselors must nevertheless increase and improve prevention efforts aimed toward women. There is no ongoing research on the efficacy of prevention strategies for women, but some survey reports, such as that done by Joyce Jackson in New Jersey, suggest that women in the minority urban populations who are at risk have a good deal of knowledge about how AIDS is spread but are nevertheless not practicing safer sex techniques—not insisting that their male partners use condoms. Interestingly, the only women showing significant behavior change are prostitutes: the Centers for Disease Control Multi-Center Prostitute Study (Centers for Disease Control, 1987) shows that 78% of prostitutes now insist that their male customers use condoms. However, even the prostitutes who make customers use condoms don't ask their boyfriends or spouses to use condoms.

Any prevention efforts targeted toward women must address the issue of why even those women knowledgeable about

AIDS don't insist upon condom use for sex. The reasons are complex, are not entirely clear, and probably are bound up in sex-role socialization and social class issues. To begin with, women in this culture are socialized to defer to men in the setting of limits for sex: Men usually determine how, when, and how often sex will occur. For a woman to suggest condom use, she must first overcome her internal barrier to setting any sexual limits. Moreover, for women sex is less likely to fulfill a pleasure function than it is to fulfill more pragmatic functions. Among these is the role of sex as a barter exchange for the financial support of a male partner. A poor woman, in particular, often cannot afford to alienate the man who supports her and her children. Many urban poor minority women at risk report fears of abandonment or even physical assault if they suggest condom use, and these women cannot simply replace a recalcitrant partner with a more compliant one that easily. Related to this is the notion of relative risk and temporally close versus temporally distant risk: If a woman balances the risk of AIDS in the future against the immediate loss of food and shelter for her and her children, safer sex loses.

A major obstacle to effective prevention for women is AIDS educators' failure to convince men of the necessity to use condoms. Safer sex messages have been in the gay male community for a number of reasons, but among these is the fact that these messages appeal more to the desire to protect oneself than the altruistic desire to protect others. That is, gay men are told to use condoms because they themselves risk AIDS from both insertive and receptive anal intercourse. Most heterosexual men have the (erroneous) impression that condoms are necessary only to protect their female partners, and thus educators are relying solely upon an altruistic motive rather than addressing the motive of self-interest. This is doubly difficult because condom use interferes with a rather rigid sexual repertoire among heterosexuals, compared with the repertoire for gay men. That is, gay men have never been as focused upon anal intercourse as a sexual mode as heterosexuals are focused upon vaginal intercourse.

Among drug users the real significance of sexual transmission has been obscured by grouping those with multiple risk factors as "IVDU" cases. In other words, a drug abusing woman who contracts AIDS is presumed to have been infected through needle use, although she may indeed have been infected through sex. Because counselors and educators tend to view all cases of

AIDS among drug users as needle-related, they underemphasize the role of sexual transmission to the very population in which they would like to change sexual habits.

It has been particularly difficult for (mostly) White professionals in the health care field to reach minority populations in an effective way. These groups often have grave mistrust of a White bureaucracy, often based upon many years of negative experiences with hospitals, social service agencies, and so forth. For example, counselors at New Jersey's AIDS service organization, the Hyacinth Foundation, are frequently asked to respond to questions from Black audiences about whether AIDS itself is a plot by the United States government to eradicate Blacks. Stories are common, both in New Jersey and New York, about health care workers being assaulted in minority communities while attempting to do prevention work handing out condoms.

As mentioned before, the impression that AIDS is associated with multiple sexual partners works against prevention efforts with women in two ways. First, it lulls some women into a false sense of security. Second, to most heterosexuals, male and female, "multiple sexual partners" translates into the pejorative term "promiscuity." This means that a woman who asks a man to use a condom is implying either that she has been promiscuous or that he has been. And finally, it is sometimes difficult for women to ask men to use condoms because women have been socialized to protect their male partners emotionally. For example, some women say they can't ask their partners to use condoms for fear of hurting their feelings; these women truly are prepared to die for love.

What, then, constitutes effective prevention strategies for women? First, on an organizational level, target prevention for the group that needs it most: inner city minority women of childbearing age. Prevention work will most effectively be done by people indigenous to the community and, for most women, by another woman. Race, class, language, and age must be considered in designing prevention strategies.

Second, construct interventions that realistically take into account the roles that sex plays in women's lives. The gay male community's emphasis upon "eroticizing safe sex," for example, is not particularly relevant to most women. What is more effective are, for example, techniques such as role-playing that help women learn how to broach the subject of condom use to their partner, or small, women-only group discussions during which participants can share feelings, fears, and successful prevention methods.

Third, convey information relevant to women, not gay men. Women need to be told that AIDS is most frequently transmitted among heterosexuals in long-term partnerships, not through multiple partners. They should be told that becoming infected can frequently take years of multiple exposures, to combat the hopeless attitude that "If I'm going to get it from him, I've already gotten it, so why start safe sex now?" Emphasize the risk from vaginal and anal sex—it is questionable whether oral sex is a vector of transmission. One is more likely to effect behavior change if one asks for change in one or two behaviors, not a whole laundry list of "possible safe" or "probably safe" behaviors. Although it is most cautious to suggest using two barriers (e.g., condoms and foam, or condoms and a diaphragm), it is also important to be realistic. Counselors at the Hyacinth Foundation tell women that if they are completely unsuccessful at getting their partners to use condoms, that other barrier methods that contain the spermicidal agent nonoxynol-9 are probably better than nothing.

Finally, target heterosexual men, not women. Here, at least two methods are important, besides the altruistic appeal to men to protect the ones they love. First, it is important to convince heterosexual men that they, too, are at risk from vaginal intercourse without a condom; it is clear that, though female to male sexual transmission may be relatively rare, it does exist. Second, one must try to get heterosexual men to change the ingrained mind-set that sex that does not include penetration of and ejaculation into a vagina (or anus) is not "real" sex. This, of course, is difficult, to say the least.

Counseling HIV-Infected Women

One of the first things a counselor must remember in dealing with HIV-infected women is that few women suspect that they are antibody positive, or infected, and that few doctors detect HIV infection, unless the woman is an intravenous drug user or reports that she is the partner of someone in a risk group. As data show, many women do not know the risk status of the men with whom they are involved. In fact, a survey of heterosexual men and women in the "general population" indicated that most women rely on simply asking their male sexual partners about risk status as their primary mode of AIDS prevention, and that approximately 50% of men said that they would lie about risk status or even antibody status in order to have sex with a woman. Thus counselors must play the unwelcome role of being the person to question risk for AIDS. Frequently the women most concerned about AIDS are the ones least likely to be at risk—middle-class women who are already somewhat phobic about sex—whereas those most at risk are also most likely to be in denial. Kathy, for example, was a middle-class woman who had a past history of intravenous drug use but who had been "clean" for 5 years. She and her husband—who knew of her past drug history—planned to have a child, and Kathy's denial regarding AIDS was so extreme that in all her medical visits to gynecologists and obstetricians she never mentioned her drug history and never asked to be tested. Finally, close to the end of her first trimester of pregnancy, her physician tested her for HIV antibodies as part of a battery of tests, and her test results were positive. Even then, the counseling she received all focused upon the odds of her baby being born infected. When she came to see a counselor, the counselor was the first person to tell her the unpleasant news that her odds of leaving her child an orphan were greater than her odds of bearing an infected baby. Despite learning of her antibody positive status, her denial was so great that it had simply not occurred to her that she might get sick and die. Thus often the most useful function a counselor can serve is to be informed about AIDS and break through clients' ignorance or denial, an ignorance or denial that health care providers may match or reinforce.

It is important for counselors to be aware that HIV-infected women are, of all persons with AIDS, perhaps the most isolated, least supported, and least cohesive group. For example, gay men who are HIV-infected have a tremendous community of support; even IVDU men who are HIV-infected have a shared bond, that of being drug users or former drug users. Because of the relatively small number of women with AIDS and because of the diversity of ways in which women can become infected with AIDS, women often find themselves most alone and feel most stigmatized. And indeed, they probably are. Partly because the level of infection is so high in the gay community, seropositive gay men can still find sexual or romantic partners. This is not true of infected women: A woman who finds herself with HIV is not likely to find another sexual or romantic partner unless she already has one or is prepared to lie. So it is not surprising that women, even more than men, feel that their lives have ended once they are infected. Group support is important for all people with AIDS; it is even more important for women. But counselors may have a hard time finding support groups for women outside of large urban areas. In these situations, it is probably helpful for counselors to try to connect women with AIDS with each other even on a one-to-one basis.

Women with AIDS are also even more likely than many others to blame themselves and be consumed with guilt and self-hatred about their infection. The fact that AIDS is associated with sex and drugs makes self-blame likely for all HIV-infected people; for women, this self-blame becomes an overlay on the cultural messages they have already received about "good girl" versus "bad girl." The self-blame reaches an almost unbearable level when children are involved. HIV-infected women with healthy children feel guilt about leaving these children behind, and women who bear infected children feel responsibility for infecting their own babies. Often, counseling must focus almost exclusively on these issues of self-hatred and blame. One of the most useful things a counselor might do for a women with AIDS could be to help her forgive herself before she dies.

Counseling with women who are HIV-infected must be pragmatic as well. Women with AIDS are likely to be poor and to be minority group members. Especially if they have children, their social service needs are many and their resources few. Counselors must be prepared to be advocates for them and to help them obtain whatever governmental entitlements they can. Counselors working with HIV-infected women may find that simple needs for housing, food, and appropriate medical care are far more important than psychological issues. Some of the social service needs these women have will involve helping them prepare to leave their children behind and to find proper homes for them. Because good foster care or adoptive care is difficult to find for these children, counselors must also help an HIV-infected woman make use of extended family networks or other support systems within her community.

It can be particularly difficult for counselors to handle their countertransferencial feelings when dealing with HIV-infected women. For example, it is easy to pass judgment upon an infected woman who chooses to carry a pregnancy to term, making it particularly important for the counselor to examine his or her own negative reaction to this. Speaking personally, as a woman who is a mother of a small child, it has been almost unbearably painful to work with HIV-infected women with children, especially when those children themselves are infected. Overidentification with the client is easy, and it is almost a requirement of this kind of counseling that the counselor be in therapy or a professional peer support group of some kind. As the death and dying counselor, Stephen Levine, said, this work requires nothing less than therapists or counselors being able to keep their heart open in hell.

References

Brooks-Gunn, J., Boyer, C.B., & Hine, K. (1988). Preventing HIV infection and AIDS in children and adolescents: Behavioral research and intervention strategies. *American Psychologist, 43*, 958–964.

Centers for Disease Control. (1987, April 17). Antibody to human immunodeficiency virus in female prostitutes. *Journal of the American Medical Association, 257*, 2011–2013.

Cohen, J., Hauer, L.B., Poole, L.E., & Wofsy, C.B. (1987). *Sexual and other practices and risk of HIV infection in a cohort of 450 sexually active women in San Francisco.* Paper presented to the III International Conference on AIDS, Washington, DC.

Fischl, M.A., Dickinson, G., Scott, G., Klimas, N., Fletcher, M.A., & Parks, W. (1987, February 6). Evaluation of heterosexual partners, children, and household contacts of adults with AIDS. *Journal of the American Medical Association, 257*, 640–644.

Friedland, G. (1987). Unpublished paper. New Jersey Department of Health.

Guinan, M.E., & Hardy, A.M. (1987, April 17). Epidemiology of AIDS in women in the United States, 1981 through 1986. *Journal of the American Medical Association, 257*, 2039–2042.

Hardy, A.M., & Guinan, M.E. (1987). *AIDS in women in the United States.* Paper presented to the III International Conference on AIDS, Washington, DC.

Kristal, A. (1986). The impact of the acquired immunodeficiency syndrome on patterns of premature death in New York City. *Journal of the American Medical Association, 255*, 2306–2310.

Landesman, S., Minkoff, H., Holman, S., McCalia, S., & Sijin, O. (1987, November 20). Serosurvey of human immunodeficiency virus infection in participants. *Journal of the American Medical Association, 258*, 2701–2703.

Padian, N., Marquis, L., Francis, D.P., Anderson, R.E., Rutherford, G., O'Malley, P., & Winkelstein, W. (1987, August 14). Male-to-female transmission of human immunodeficiency virus. *Journal of the American Medical Association*, *258*, 788–790.

Peckham, C.S., Sentuvia, Y.D., & Ades, A.E. (1987). Obstetric and perinatal consequences of human immunodeficiency virus (HIV) infection: A review. *British Journal of Obstetrics and Gynecology*, *94*, 403–407.

Chapter 5

SPECIAL NEEDS OF TODAY'S ADOLESCENTS

Barbara R. Slater

The current AIDS crisis affects all society, with particular meaning for youth. Counselors working with youth who are affected by AIDS need to look at the dual educative and therapeutic aspects in their ongoing work. Almost all children and adolescents attend school and, therefore, schools are drawn into the heart of the crisis as major vehicles for providing current, accurate information on HIV characteristics, transmission, and prevention. Counselors working with youth need to consider schools as a focus of educative programs, with strong liaison ties to other organizations that have specialized AIDS-related services.

Because other chapters in this text and other experts in the field have written extensively about the history and current status of information about AIDS, this chapter will not attend to these issues but, rather, will address the specific needs of youth. According to October, 1988, data from the Centers for Disease Control (1988b), 75,768 persons have been documented as having AIDS, 1,202 of them are younger than 13 and 305 are between ages 13 and 20. The CDC anticipates as many as 3,000 diagnosed childhood AIDS cases (under age 13) in the United States by 1991 (CDC, 1988a) and others feel that this figure may reach 20,000 (Diamond & Cohen, 1987; Oleske, 1987). The number of adolescents with AIDS is comparatively small but it is doubling each year (Brooks-Gunn, Boyer, & Hein, 1988). Counselors will be working with these young persons as they progress through childhood and into adolescence, should they survive that long.

Minority youth are differentially affected by AIDS so that counselors will want to consider the specific needs of minority youth in their work. The CDC (1988b) reported that as of October 18, 1988, among those under age 20, White children and youth accounted for 28% (425) of the cases of AIDS, Black children and youth for 49% (735), Hispanic children and youth for 22% (330), and others for 1% (14). These figures clearly do not reflect overall population characteristics.

We have no estimate of how many other young persons there are who are HIV-infected (seropositive) but undetected, all of them carriers of the HIV. In addition to those children and youth who have AIDS, those who have AIDS-related complex (ARC) and demonstrate some AIDS-related symptoms and those who are HIV-positive but asymptomatic also must be considered. Although many lay persons lump these categories together, the needs of the affected persons are different. Still another category is the "worried well," youth who are not infected but who are extremely anxious because they engage in high-risk behaviors or fear contracting AIDS through non-high-risk behaviors.

AIDS is presently an incurable, fatal disease, so that the only means of eliminating it lies in prevention, and prevention requires abstention, safer practices in sexual and IV drug behaviors, or monogamous, nonrisk behavior relationships. In order for this to occur, all youth must be reached before they engage in high-risk behaviors or our efforts will be in vain. From another perspective, youth who already are HIV-infected require enormous amounts of support and assistance in facing the grim realities of the future.

What Do Adolescents Think, Believe, and Know And Why Is This So?

The Period of Exploration and Invulnerability

Adolescence is characterized by the need to explore many facets of life and by a sense of invulnerability, the "it happens to others, not to me" approach to life. This combination of experimentation and perceived invulnerability makes it more likely that adolescents will engage in high-risk behaviors. Kotulak (1987) noted that "doctors now refer to the new morbidity of adolescents, recognizing that risk-taking behavior presents extremely grave health threats to teenagers" (p. 2). The Institute of Medicine and the National Academy of Sciences (1986) also noted the need to stress prevention with adolescents because of sex and drug experimentation. An interesting aspect in the adolescent's striving for adulthood is the conflict between the need for individuality and the need to behave in a manner consistent with one's peers. In order to influence young persons so that they engage in lower risk behaviors, counselors need to reach them before peer group influence has become strong and in a manner so as to encourage healthful individuality. Otherwise, their attempts to prove their individuality may result in increased risk taking.

An additional problem, often based in myth, is the attitude that, "I know how to be safe." When one looks at data on sexual behavior and on contraception use among sexually active youth, the danger of this attitude becomes obvious. In a summary of facts about AIDS and teenagers (Select Committee on Children, Youth, and Families, undated), it was reported that from 33% to 55% of teenagers surveyed in San Francisco and Massachusetts indicated that they were not worried about contracting AIDS and, in Massachusetts, only 15% of the 70% who were sexually active indicated that they had changed sexual behaviors because of concern about AIDS. The Center for Population Options (1987) reported that of sexually active, unmarried 15- to 19-year-old women, only 34% used any birth control method consistently and, of those who did use birth control, only 22% insisted their partners use condoms, leaving 78% using contraceptives offering no HIV protection. Considering the fact that over one half of all 15- to 19-year-olds (Shafer, 1987) and 70% (women) to 80% (men) of all 20-year-olds (Center for Population Options) are sexually active, the myth of knowing how to have safe sex is a dangerous one that all counselors must address.

Cultural Differences

As noted, minority youth are differentially affected by AIDS. Although cultural characteristics and attitudes vary from locale to locale, it is useful to examine some of the factors that may result in a potential higher risk for Black and Hispanic youth, because it has been documented that current informational materials are not effective with these youth (DiClemente, Boyer, & Morales, 1988; Fullilove, 1988; Mays & Cochran, 1987).

Many minority young men are burdened with the attitude that safer sex implies a fault in masculinity such as homosexuality or infection with a sexually transmitted disease and therefore feel that they cannot use contraceptives or maintain a monogamous relationship. Abstention might be seen as an admission that something "is wrong." Similarly, minority young women often feel that they cannot insist upon safer sex because it would be a direct insult to their partners' masculinity and health status. Such insistence could well result in ostracism for some young women because it is considered unacceptable for a woman to have knowledge about sexuality or question a man (Mays & Cochran, 1988). In a society that encourages early sexuality and "couple" behavior, this would be particularly problematic for poor or neglected youth who experience a strong need for affection and social acceptance. Because homophobia is often strong in some Black and Hispanic cultures (Peterson & Marin, 1988), the fear of being labeled gay if one is not actively heterosexual is an additional block to low-risk behavior. Seeking help is also an issue among many minority cultures, making it difficult for youth to obtain information or assistance because they might be seen as weak or as going against cultural tradition.

A similar problem may exist in Black and Hispanic attitudes toward drug abuse among urban youth. Peer pressure and a sense of hopelessness among poor youth can result in IV drug abuse in order to maintain distance from the constant negativity of life or to maintain status in the subculture. The "macho" attitude of the proof of manliness through drug abuse and the need of many young women to comply with their partners' demands further increase the risk of destructive behavior. Certainly counselors need to consider the possible effects of membership in a minority culture on both sexual and drug abuse behaviors among their clients.

Lack of Effectiveness of Educative Efforts

It has been established that current AIDS education programs are not reaching adolescents (DiClemente, Boyer, & Morales, 1988; Dictemente, Zorn, & Temoshok, 1986; Fullilove, 1988; Shafer, 1987; Slater, 1988b, in press). Surveys and studies of adolescents (Brown & Fritz, 1987; DiClemente, Boyer, & Morales, 1988; Dictemente, Zorn, & Temoshok, 1986; Shafer, 1987) have highlighted the lack of information that adolescents possess about causes and prevention of AIDS, particularly among minority youth. The schools, which "have become a bastion of AIDS misconceptions and irrational fears" (Horan & Sherman, 1988) are ill prepared to develop and implement effective educational programs (Slater, 1988b). Yet they are the single means of reaching almost all youth. Although most adults seem to believe that youth need to be informed of the dangers of AIDS, there is great reluctance to address issues of drugs, sexuality, and homosexuality directly. Until appropriate school programs can be implemented, AIDS education will take place in a piecemeal fashion. Counselors need to direct efforts toward educating the educators and the lay public about the need for powerful, school-based programs on prevention of AIDS.

What is needed to make educative programs, regardless of where they are located, more effective?

1. They must gear materials to the developmental level of target youth. Because of adolescents' impulsiveness, experimentation, and a lack of well-developed abstract skills, materials need to be concrete and to provide ideas and techniques that permit youth to delay the immediate gratification of desires by highlighting real rewards for such delay and by making delay socially acceptable. As programs must reach downward in age so as to inform and influence children prior to the onset of high-risk behaviors, they must also be attentive to the age-appropriateness of materials.

2. They must provide current and accurate information about HIV characteristics, transmission, and prevention that convince youth of the severity of the crisis, and they must offer viable alternatives to high-risk behavior. Because information alone seldom results in behavioral change (Flora & Thorensen, 1988; Melton, 1988a), program materials must provide compelling case studies and peer-generated materials such as videos, posters, cassettes, and so forth so as to involve the youth in the educative process. An example of an effective approach was one schoolwide contest to produce rap material about AIDS that resulted in the entire school's involvement.

3. They must use language that is understood by and relevant to youth. The majority of printed materials are written for White, middle-class adults or adolescents at a relatively high language level (Jue, 1988) and are inappropriate for large num-

bers of youth in terms of understandability and appeal. In other words, they do not capture and hold the interest of the target group. Comic book material such as *Hero Comix Group: Andrea and Lisa* (Health Education Resource Organization, 1987) does seem to be a viable approach. As so clearly set forth by Mays and Cochran (1987), minority-geared material must use appropriate vernacular in describing sexual and IV drug use behaviors. Materials for Hispanic youth need to be available in Spanish and English, as, for example, *When A Friend Has AIDS* (Chelsea Psychotherapy Associates, 1984), *AIDS Hotlines* (Gay Men's Health Crisis, 1986) or *Straight Talk About Sex and AIDS* (San Francisco AIDS Foundation, 1986).

4. They must address the needs of minority youth in terms of cultural attitudes, beliefs, traditions, and values. In order for this to happen, minority persons need to be involved in the development of such materials and, prior to distribution, all such materials need to be evaluated by panels of minority youth to determine relevance and appeal.

5. They must address drug abuse, sexuality, and homosexuality directly without evoking strong community resistance. This requires emphasis on protecting the lives of youth, not on encouraging behaviors that threaten the community by going against mainstream society. Youthful abstinence probably will need attention whether or not the counselor believes in its appropriateness or reality. Keep in mind that a program that has been banned or canceled cannot assist anyone.

6. They must offer treatment options or recommendations for those youth who need mental health support or treatment. This aspect of the program needs to allay anxiety and overcome resistance to seeking counseling.

Major Issues Adolescents Face

"Catching" AIDS

Contracting AIDS is a concern of many youth, although not as many as one would expect. Among those with whom counselors will have contact are the "worried well." Because these youth often are not engaging in high-risk behaviors, counselors need to assess the reality factor in each case. With young gay men, because of the possibility of transmission of the HIV through anal or oral sex, anxiety is realistic unless a young man has never engaged in these sexual behaviors and the youth intends to follow safer sex practices. IV drug abusing youth also have realistic anxiety. If a youth is at low risk, AIDS-related counseling needs to attend to overall high anxiety aspects of personality development, with concomitant provision of clear information on HIV transmission and prevention and with reality testing of the interface between actual behaviors and risk factors. One will usually find evidence of many other anxieties in these youth.

Passive transfer, contracting the HIV without engaging in any known high-risk behaviors, has both realistic and unrealistic aspects. Among the most realistic factors are pre/perinatal transfer from the infected mother to the infant, and blood or blood factor transfer through transfusion prior to the initiation of blood testing. With an unknown latency between infection and onset, there certainly are youngsters who have become infected but are asymptomatic. If there is a strong possibility of infection, (e.g., a high-risk mother, transfusion after a trauma, hemophilia, etc.), this author believes that it is wise to recommend and to assist in obtaining anonymous (not confidential) antibody testing, with a repetition of the testing in 6 months if the first results are negative. It should be noted that others do not espouse this point of view, and some feel that the dangers to the client of testing outweigh the benefits (Coates, Stall, Kegeles, Lo, Morin, & McKusick, 1988). Of course, should a positive result be obtained and verified through additional evaluation, counseling will take on an entirely different character and require intensive work. A negative result can be used to reassure, except in rare circumstances (Goldblum & Marks, 1988), *provided* that there have been no high-risk aspects for several years and that no high-risk behaviors are engaged in from the time of the original antibody test.

Unrealistic factors are usually based in the myths promulgated widely in society as to the dangers related to casual or daily living contact. Although the literature has made it clear that AIDS is not transmitted by insects, by toilet seats, by physical, nonsexual touch, by sharing eating implements, by sharing the same classroom, by living together, and so forth (Centers for Disease Control, 1986; Committee on Infectious Diseases, 1987; Fischl, Dickinson, Scott, Klimas, Fletcher, & Parks, 1987; Friedland et al., 1986; Friedland et al., 1987; Koop, 1986; Slater, 1988b), these myths continue to abound. As in the case of the low-risk, "worried well" youth, information developed specifically for youth, such as *AIDS: You Can't Catch It Holding Hands* (de Saint Phalle, 1987) and *Understanding and Preventing AIDS: A Guide for Young People* (Colman, 1988) can be of assistance in developing healthier attitudes.

Active transfer, becoming HIV-infected through engaging in high-risk sexual or IV drug abuse behaviors, is of great concern to a number of youth, both gay and heterosexual. Among all of the clusters of persons vulnerable to HIV infection, including everyone except those who are celibate, who do not abuse drugs, or who are in monogamous, nonrisk relationships, the most distinctive behavioral changes have been made in the gay community. Because of intensive educative campaigns, gay youth who have been able to benefit from these efforts are now more likely to follow safer sex practices, thus reducing risk. However, counselors will have their hands full working with all youth who endanger themselves through risky behavior, including gay youth who have been unable to avail themselves of information about more reasonable behaviors, IV drug abusers, and heterosexual youth who have had sexual or IV drug contact with infected persons.

The Emotional Impact of AIDS

Another issue young people face is the emotional impact associated with knowing or hearing about others who are HIV-positive, who have AIDS, or who have died of AIDS-related opportunistic diseases. As a result of the long latency period, it is less likely that adolescents will personally know persons with AIDS. However, counselors must be prepared to deal directly with this issue when it does occur. Youth who know of a peer who is HIV-positive will need to resolve the possible fear of contracting AIDS from that peer, the shock of perceiving the peer in a different light, and the issues surrounding death and dying. If the affected person is a relative, particularly one close to the youth, the same issues will evolve but with death and dying aspects heightened. In addition, if the youth has not had a good relationship with the affected person, guilt over not having behaved in an "appropriate" manner may be felt.

When youth become aware of a person with AIDS who is known to them in a way not mentioned above, the reaction can vary markedly from horror and fear, as in the case of a well-liked teacher, to curiosity, as in the case of a well-known public figure. The more attention given by the media, as in the case of an actor or athlete, the more likely that curiosity will be present without extreme fear. If the noted person has died, stronger feelings are apt to be evoked.

In any of the situations noted, strong reassurance and support are called for. If the youth has incorrect information leading to the escalation of anxiety and fear, information is also warranted. It is strongly suggested that counselors, and others, be prepared to present programs to the youth and staff of a school, church, social/athletic organization, or any other formal program should a person who is connected to that setting die of AIDS-related conditions or become incapacitated because of AIDS. If the affected person continues normal activities, then youth may need to be encouraged to treat the individual as they would anyone else if problems about AIDS arise.

Homophobia and AIDS

Homophobia as it relates to AIDS affects many gay and lesbian youth. Homophobia, defined as "the recognized or unrecognized fear or hatred of homosexuality or homosexuals that is present in both heterosexuals and homosexuals" (Slater, 1988a, p. 227), has been attached strongly to AIDS. In turn, this has resulted in an escalation of prejudice against, rejection of, harassment of, and attack on gays and persons suspected of being gay (Altman, 1986; Berrill, 1985), thus increasing young gay men's fears of coming out.

Although it is clear that gay men are the highest risk group and young men must face this fact, it is equally clear that being gay does not mean that one is infected. Counselors will need to work intensively to repair the damaged self-concept of many young gays who have come to see themselves as degenerates or evil because of society's messages. These negative self-perceptions make it extremely difficult for young gay men to seek either information or counseling because of a fear of being seen as "sick" by the counselor.

Of extreme concern is the pain closeted gay youth face who are HIV-positive and who must deal simultaneously with a life-threatening condition and coming out to important others. These youth require even more massive support and assistance than youth who are already open to family and friends. Bibliotherapy is useful, particularly the form that provides materials for reading and then uses the obtained information as a springboard for therapy discussion. Because of the difficulty of youth in obtaining appropriate material on coming out and on AIDS, both from a cost perspective and from the perspective of having to enter a gay/lesbian bookstore to obtain these materials, it is recommended that counselors develop libraries of books, pamphlets, articles, audiotapes and other materials for loan purposes. Public and school libraries are sadly lacking in current, relevant books. As has been noted, the gay community has been most effective in developing resources related to AIDS. It is, therefore, recommended that counselors maintain strong liaisons to gay organizations in their area so that direct referral of youth to the most appropriate supportive programs and resources can be accomplished quickly and easily.

Therapy Aspects

Although many aspects of therapy apply across a variety of youth, it is useful to explore aspects that are particularly relevant to specific populations. Among these populations are adolescents in general; high-risk adolescents; and adolescents who are HIV-positive, who have ARC, or who have AIDS.

Youth in General

In counseling all youth, AIDS ought to be an integral part of the process so as to reduce the potential for risky behaviors. Obviously this aspect of counseling can take place only in the overall context of counseling and cannot be allowed to interfere with crisis situations. Often youth have not had the opportunity to discuss their fears, thoughts, and attitudes about AIDS and so will welcome a safe and open ground for such discussion. Certainly the provision of information about disease characteristics and prevention can be accomplished in a straightforward manner, taking into consideration those aspects noted in the section of educational efforts. Time needs to be spent on the demystification of AIDS so that youth can develop a more realistic view of AIDS.

Anxieties related to AIDS most probably will need to be integrated into the overall fabric of anxiety characteristics in the individual counselee. As has been noted, low-risk, "worried well" youth frequently are high-anxiety individuals, so the counselor will be working with anxiety as an overall personality factor.

In order to effect low-risk behaviors, counselors may wish to consider what means will be most effective to build confidence in the self while concomitantly lowering the sense of invulnerability. As an aspect of impulse control, it also will be helpful to assist in the development of a sense of being able to deal effectively with one's needs in a reasonable and safe manner. Part of the movement toward safer behaviors is the building of a network of peers and adults upon whom the youth can rely when he or she needs to talk about intimate issues, and a counselor can implement this growth process.

High-Risk Youth: IV Drug Abusers

All of the ideas presented in the previous section are useful in working with IV drug-abusing youth. In addition, preparation for entry into a drug program is essential, as it is unlikely that a drug-abusing youth will be able to give up a drug habit without the intensive support provided by such specific-intent programs. It is common for these youth to experience isolation and feelings of unworthiness so that counselors will need to work toward alleviation of the negative self-image and building up of an appropriate support network if the youth is to be able to even consider cessation of self-destructive behaviors associated with drug abuse.

High-Risk Youth: Gay Men and Lesbians

Again, all of the ideas noted in the section of youth in general are useful. In addition, treatment of gayness or lesbianism as an essentially normal variation of life is critical. If this is to succeed, it must take place in a low-homophobic counseling environment so as to permit the development of trust in a safe adult. Obviously, because so many youth are in the pre-coming-out process either to themselves or to others, counselors must present a low-homophobic profile to all youth. A counselor never knows when the youth sitting in the other chair is gay or lesbian. If the young person is aware that homosexuality is not seen as bad, evil, or sick, it then becomes possible to explore his or her orientation and to come out to the counselor.

Once it has been established that the client is gay or lesbian, issues related to homosexuality and AIDS can become a part of the counseling. It needs to be clearly stated here that a gay or lesbian status should never be considered to be the problem. In needs equal emphasis that being gay or lesbian has its own difficulties because of the typical negative messages transmitted throughout society about homosexuality. Although a young gay man or lesbian most certainly may have problems associated with orientation, it is the beliefs and attitudes, not the orientation, that cause difficulties. Provision of information related to being gay or lesbian ought to include objective and accurate facts about homosexuality, coming-out processes, developmental stages, forming relationships, and the development of support networks in the community (Slater, 1988a). Once again, bibliotherapy is one of the most useful educative aspects of counseling with lesbian and gay youth.

Although lesbians are discussed here, they are in the next lowest risk group following non-drug users, sexual celibates, and those in long-term monogamous and nonrisk behavior relationships. However, it is important to communicate to young lesbians that they are not protected from AIDS and to discuss with them how the HIV can be transmitted to lesbians who have partners who are IV drug abusers, are bisexual, or have had relationships with high-risk lesbians. The rather down-to-earth saying that one goes to bed with everyone with whom the partner has had sexual or IV drug abuse contact is accurate. Safer sex practices ought to become a part of counseling with young lesbians.

Clients who are young gay men face many more frightening possibilities than do most lesbians. Harassment and violence have been more strongly directed against gays, although it is clear that lesbians also experience both. The possibility of being harmed because of one's orientation typically leads to anxiety, fear, and anger. All of these reactions need to be dealt with in the counseling environment, which becomes a safe place to ventilate and then work through the anger and frustration associated with society's inappropriate reactions toward the youth. Gay youth who come out often face rejection by peers, family, and important others. Sometimes this rejection is temporary, but it can be permanent. This needs to be taken into consideration when one is assisting youth in determining whether to come out and, if so, to whom, when, and how. A counselor must be realistic in discussing possible reactions of key persons in the youth's life. AIDS has added another dimension to this issue because so many individuals associate homosexuality and AIDS in a manner that escalates negativity toward the target youth. Counselors ought to be prepared to act as major support persons in the lives of their coming-out youths and to devote serious efforts toward alleviating the negative self-concepts that develop as a result of rejection. The concept of a second chance family, originally developed by Malamud and Machover (1965), can be brought into play here as the youth is encouraged to develop a supportive network or current family similar to an ideal family.

Providing information about safer gay sexual practices is, of course, a part of any counseling with young gays, although it may not be able to be brought into the situation until more pressing issues have been dealt with, at least to the extent that crises have been reduced to a tolerable level. This information must be concrete and graphic if it is to be of use. As previously noted, open young gay men already may have benefited from the educative materials developed by gay organizations so that counselors can build upon that knowledge. In the case of coming-out or closeted youth, the counselor may become the key figure in information development. It is suggested that counselors follow the lead of clients in the use of sexually relevant terms, concepts, and phrases. This means that counselors must carefully inspect their own biases and comfort related to sexuality before attempting to discuss sexuality with clients, particularly with gay youth. If the client has not developed a language, then it will be necessary for the counselor to assist in the development of a working vocabulary before the process can proceed further.

Youth Who Have AIDS, Who Have ARC, or Who Are HIV-Positive

Primary to treatment is the provision of an accepting, non-fearful atmosphere in which the young person can receive the massive support and caring necessary for infected individuals. In order to handle this, counselors will have to examine their own responses to AIDS and, perhaps, receive assistance in attaining a comfortable stance. Although all persons ought to respect and fear the HIV, it is not necessary to fear HIV transmission from a client.

Development of an understanding of the meaning of being HIV-positive, of having ARC, or of having AIDS requires the

naked truth as much as the individual counselee can handle it.
Knowing that one is infected results in a new identity crisis
following relatively close on the heels of the overall adolescent
identity crisis and, possibly, redefinition of the self as gay. Added
to this is the issue of rejection that has already been discussed.

With HIV-positive youth, assistance in realistically planning for an unknown future and living in short blocks of time,
in living as healthful a life style as is possible, in dealing with
deadly stresses compounded by important persons in the youth's
life, and in accepting a basically unacceptable future become
the core of counseling. Because there is no clear knowledge as
to how long a person can be HIV-positive without developing
symptoms or what proportion of HIV-infected individuals will
develop full-blown AIDS, the anxiety and despair the knowledge of an HIV-positive status engenders is overwhelming. Stages
of denial, anger, and mourning will need to be endured. Impulsive acting up, possibly sexually, will also have to be dealt
with quite directly in terms of its meaning and the likelihood
of HIV transmission to others.

Counselors will need to consider the legal and ethical issues
of confidentiality versus the need to inform parents or the need
to warn endangered sexual or IV drug abuse partners. Because
this is a new issue, there are no specific guidelines or legal con-
clusions for youth at this time and counselors will have to continue
to consult the literature for emerging information. Generally,
parents of minority age youth have the right, under public law,
of access to school records so that school counselors and psychologists would need to consider the ramifications of AIDS information that appear in any records. In cases where counselees
are guaranteed confidentiality under federal regulations covering
certain drug rehabilitation programs and in states that permit
adolescents access to health care for sexually transmitted diseases
without parent consent or knowledge, there may be clearer guidelines. In terms of the need to warn, Melton (1988b) pointed out
that the Tarasoff decision was primarily related to intent or certainty of harm and that unprotected sex or IV drug abuse does
not have such certainty. He did, however, note that states can
legislate requirements to release confidential data as new legislation or connected to principles of public health law. Because it
has not yet been subjected to litigation, we to not know if a parent
or infected sex/IV drug abuse partner can bring successful legal
action against a counselor who has maintained confidentiality related to AIDS information. It is clear that counselors need to

ascertain the legal and ethical situation in their locales and to apprise counselees of the limits of confidentiality that exist or that the counselor assumes exist. The issues of legal or ethical responsibility need to be considered apart from the counselor's estimate of the desirability of bringing others who may be affected by the counselee's status into the counseling situation.

For youth with AIDS, one of the primary responsibilities of the counselor will be leading the youth through the stages of initial crisis, early adjustment or the transitional stage, acceptance or the deficiency stage, and preparation for death (Nichols & Ostrow, 1984). Stein and Cohen (1986) effectively discussed therapy related to these stages. Loss, of three varieties that can be labeled as "loss of control, loss of the sense of identity, and loss of relationships" (Hidalgo, Peterson, & Woodman, 1985, p. 75), will also consume considerable counseling time. Because of the deterioration typical of AIDS, work will need to be rapid if it is to help the youth, and the counselor will need to be prepared to work with a person who changes rapidly in terms of physical and mental functioning. Dealing with potential suicide and sexual acting up may also become part of the treatment.

Because rejection is so typical, the counselor may become the client's emotional parent, lover, friend, and educator and, therefore, will experience enormous drains of energy and burdens of responsibility. It is strongly recommended that any counselor working with AIDS youth develop a strong professional and personal support network so that issues related to the counseling can be resolved. Counselors also ought to anticipate that they will be with the youth until he or she dies so that preparation for the anticipated deterioration and impending death must be undertaken. It is recommended that focus be placed on developing new support systems or strengthening already existing support systems for the youth. Where family are available, including the affectional partners of the youth, counseling will need to include these important persons.

Counseling Techniques

Counseling techniques related to AIDS should be integrated into most theoretical frameworks with some necessary changes to account for the unique characteristics of AIDS counseling. Counselors may need to alter their theoretical perspectives to be more responsive to the severity of the condition, the need to provide more nurturance and support than is typical in most counseling situations, and the need to provide more specific information than is typical. Any model that depends upon a long period of time to effect change cannot be used effectively because of the usual truncation of the life span. Counseling with youth affected by the HIV does need to contain both educative and directive aspects in addition to more traditional aspects.

The role-model of nonbias is critical, as has already been discussed. It may be that the counselor is the first or only person to accept the infected youth, thus the role-modeling aspect of counseling serves two purposes: reassurance that the youth is an acceptable human being and provision of the impetus for developing a more positive self-concept. In addition to the role-model aspect, massive support and nurturing are necessary if the youth is to face the specter of death connected to AIDS.

The involvement of family members and, in the case of older youth, of important others such as intimate friends or lovers, in the counseling process is particularly useful in the overall therapeutic plan. This involvement permits others to interact in a more helpful manner with the infected youth and to understand more fully what is occurring. It also expands the support network so as to distribute responsibility for the young person more equally. Obviously this can only happen if others are available and amenable to working with the counselor and counselee. Otherwise, counseling may have to focus on the sense of aloneness or rejection.

Two techniques that have proven to be especially useful are group, including dyadic, counseling and bibliotherapy. Group approaches allow for the development of a broader network and discussion of issues intimately involved with AIDS. As all members of the group share a core trauma, discussion can be more open and support can be more intensive than can usually occur in individual counseling. Bibliotherapy has both educative and therapeutic aspects and can be an integral part of ongoing counseling. As has been mentioned, the counselor will need to develop a library of appropriate materials for loan to clients.

Implications for Practitioners

In order to work effectively with youth who are HIV-infected, counselors have a number of needs to consider. Although the following list is not exhaustive, each item on it has been discussed in the text and is an important consideration.

1. Counselors need to be well informed; to have at their command the most accurate, current data.
2. Counselors need to explore their own biases and fears. A counselor cannot work with HIV-positive youth if he or she is fearful or highly anxious, and cannot work with gays or lesbians if he or she is homophobic.
3. Counselors need to be able to communicate directly and effectively with youth, especially about sexuality. This is particularly important in working with minority youth and with economically disadvantaged youth.
4. Counselors need to be willing to turn to authorities on AIDS and to community resources with a sense of comfort.
5. Counselors need to be willing to include educative aspects within the counseling framework and to be directive when it is called for in relation to information and high-risk behaviors.
6. Counselors need to be able to offer support and caring beyond that typically anticipated within a counseling situation.
7. Counselors need to be able to tolerate the probability of the death of their clients without withdrawing needed caring. This draws enormously on the energy of the counselor and requires that the counselor have a professional and personal support network to work out the draining issues related to counseling a youth with AIDS.
8. Counselors need to be willing to share with others any aspect of counseling that either works or fails to work so as to develop a better body of information and techniques that can be used to counsel youth who are HIV-positive.
9. Counselors need to be creative and innovative in developing new approaches to counseling that are more suitable for the target group. This requires a solid grounding in theory and a confidence in their ability to move into new territory. Obviously, a drastically different approach ought to be discussed with respected peers prior to initiation.
10. Counselors need to recognize and accept the imperfect aspect of their knowledge of this crisis as well as the

ability of therapy as we know it to be effective, and be willing to move ahead even with this knowledge.

Summary

Work with HIV-positive youth is compounded by the tendency of adolescents to explore sexuality and to see themselves as invulnerable. It is clear that current educative efforts are not effective, particularly with minority youth. Youth face issues of the "worried well," fear of passive or active transmission of the HIV, the emotional impact of AIDS, and homophobia. Counseling must address the needs of youth in general, IV drug abusing youth, gay and lesbian youth, and youth who are HIV-positive and nonsymptomatic, who have AIDS-related complex, or who have full-blown AIDS. Although there is no preference of one technique over another, speed is essential, the educative aspects must be addressed, the counselor must provide massive support, and the counselor must have an adequate support system.

References

Altman, D. (1986). *AIDS in the mind of America*. Garden City, NY: Anchor Press/Doubleday.

Berril, K. (1985). *Anti-gay violence and victimization*. New York: National Gay and Lesbian Task Force.

Brooks-Gunn, J., Boyer, C.B., & Hein, K. (1988). Preventing HIV infection and AIDS in children and adolescents. *American Psychologist, 43*(11), 958–964.

Brown, L.K., & Fritz, G.K. (1987). *Children's knowledge and attitudes about AIDS*. Poster presentation to the American Academy of Child and Adolescent Psychiatry's 39th Annual Meeting, Washington, DC.

Centers For Disease Control. (1986). Apparent transmission of human T-lymphotropic virus type III/lymphadenopathy-associated virus from a child to a mother providing health care. *Morbidity and Mortality Weekly Report, 35*, 76–79.

Centers For Disease Control. (1988a, January 29). Guidelines for effective health education to prevent the spread of AIDS. *Morbidity and Mortality Weekly Report, 37*, 1–14.

Centers For Disease Control. (1988b, July 18). *Weekly Surveillance Report*. Atlanta: Department of Health and Human Services.

Center for Population Options. (1987, April). *AIDS and adolescents*. New York: Author.

Chelsea Psychotherapy Associates. (1986). *When a friend has AIDS. . . .* New York: Author.

Coates, T.J., Stall, R.D., Kegeles, S.M., Lo, B., Morin, S.F., & McKusick, L. (1988). AIDS antibody testing: Will it stop the AIDS epidemic? Will it help people infected with HIV? *American Psychologist, 43*(11), 859–864.

Colman, W. (1988). *Understanding and preventing AIDS: A guide for young people.* Chicago: Children's Press.

Committee on Infectious Diseases. (1987). Health guidelines for the attendance in day-care and foster care settings of children infected with human immunodeficiency virus. *Pediatrics, 79*(3), 466–469.

de Saint Phalle, N. (1987). *AIDS: You can't catch it holding hands.* San Francisco: Lapis Press.

Diamond, G.W., & Cohen, H.J. (1987, December). *AIDS and developmental disabilities. Prevention update (The National Coalition on Prevention of Mental Retardation).* Silver Spring, MD: The National Coalition on Prevention of Mental Retardation.

DiClemente, R.J., Boyer, C.B., & Morales, E. (1988). Minorities and AIDS: Knowledge, attitudes and misconceptions among Black and Latino adolescents. *American Journal of Public Health, 78,* 55–57.

Dictemente, R.G., Zorn, J., & Temoshok, L. (1986). Adolescents and AIDS: A survey of knowledge, attitudes, and beliefs about AIDS in San Francisco. *Journal of Public Health, 76,* 1443–1445.

Fischl, M.A., Dickinson, G.M., Scott, C.B., Klimas, N., Fletcher, M.A., & Parks, W. (1987). Evaluation of heterosexual partners, children and household contacts of adults with AIDS. *Journal of the American Medical Association, 257,* 640–644.

Flora, J.A., & Thorensen, C.E. (1988). Reducing the risk of AIDS in adolescents. *American Psychologist, 43*(11), 965–970.

Friedland, G.H., Saltzman, B.R., Rogers, M.R., Kahl, P.A., Feiner, C., & Mayers, M.M. (1987, June). Lack of transmission of HIV infection to household contacts of AIDS patients. *Supplement to the AIDS record: III International Conference on AIDS.* Washington, DC: Bio-Data Publishers.

Friedland, G.H., Saltzman, B.R., Rogers, M.R., Kahl, P.A., Lesser, M.L., Mayers, M.M., & Klein, R.S. (1986). Lack of transmission of HTLV/LAV infection to household contacts of patients with AIDS or AIDS-related complex with oral candidiasis. *New England Journal of Medicine, 314,* 344–349.

Fullilove, R.E. (1988). Minorities and AIDS: A review of recent publications. *Multicultural Inquiry and Research on AIDS, 2,* 2–5.

Gay Men's Health Crisis, Inc. (1986). *AIDS hotline.* New York: Author.

Goldblum, P., & Marks, R. (1988). The HIV testing debate. *Focus: A Guide to AIDS Research, 3*(12), 1–3.

Health Education Resource Organization. (1987). *Hero comix group: Andrea and Lisa.* Baltimore: Author.

Hidalgo, H., Peterson, T.L., & Woodman, N.J. (Eds.). (1985). *Lesbian and gay issues; A resource manual for social workers*. Silver Spring, MD: National Association of Social Workers.

Horan, P.F., & Sherman, R.A. (1988). School psychologists and the AIDS epidemic. *Professional School Psychology, 3*(1), 33–49.

Institute of Medicine and National Academy of Sciences. (1986). *Confronting AIDS: Directions for public health, health care, and research*. Washington, DC: National Academy Press.

Jue, S. (1988, September). AIDS and cross-cultural counseling. *Focus: A Guide to AIDS Research, 3*(10), 3–4.

Koop, C.E. (1986). *The Surgeon General's report on acquired immunodeficiency syndrome*. Washington, DC: U.S. Public Health Services.

Kotulak, R. (1987). Growing up at risk (pamphlet). *Chicago Tribune*.

Malamud, D.I., & Machover, S. (1985). *Toward self-understanding: Group techniques in self-confrontation*. Springfield, IL: Charles C Thomas.

Mays, V.M., & Cochran, S.D. (1987). Acquired immunodeficiency syndrome and Black Americans. *Public Health Reports, 19*(4), 403–408.

Mays, V.M., & Cochran, S.D. (1988). Issues in the perception of AIDS risk and risk reduction activities by Black and Hispanic/Latino women. *American Psychologist, 43*(11), 949–957.

Melton, G.B. (1988a). Adolescents and prevention of AIDS. *Professional Psychology: Research and Practice, 19*(4), 403–406.

Melton, G.B. (1988b). Ethical and legal issues in AIDS-related practice. *American Psychologist, 43*(11), 941–947.

Nichols, S.E., & Ostrow, D.G. (1984). *Psychiatric implications of the acquired immunodeficiency syndrome*. Washington, DC: American Psychiatric Press.

Oleske, J. (1987). Natural history of HIV infection II. In U.S. Department of Health and Human Services, *Report of the Surgeon General's workshop on children with HIV infection and their families*. Rockville, MD: U.S. Department of Health and Human Services.

Peterson, J.L., & Marin, G. (1988). Issues in the prevention of AIDS among Black and Hispanic men. *American Psychologist, 43*(11), 871–877.

San Francisco AIDS Foundation. (1986). *Straight talk about sex and AIDS* . San Francisco: Author.

Select Committee on Children, Youth, and Families. (undated). *Fact sheet: AIDS and teenagers*. Washington, DC: U.S. House of Representatives.

Shafer, M. (1987). *Testimony prepared for the hearing of the Select Committee on Children, Youth, and Families of the U.S. House of Representatives*. Washington, DC: U.S. House of Representatives.

Slater, B.R. (1988a). Essential issues in working with lesbian and gay male youths. *Professional Psychology: Research and Practice, 19*(2), 226–235.

Slater, B.R. (1988b, August). *Pediatric AIDS in the schools: A needs survey*. Paper presented to the Annual Convention of the American Psychological Association, Atlanta. (Audio Transcripts: 191–433–88. 610 Madison St., Alexandria, VA 22314)

Slater, B.R. (in press). Anxiety about AIDS in the schools: Student, parent, and staff issues. In J. Kaufman (Ed.). *Children with AIDS: A sourcebook for professionals*. New York: Guilford.

Stein, T.S., & Cohen, C.J. (1986). *Contemporary perspectives on psychotherapy with lesbians and gay men*. New York: Plenum Medical Book Company.

Chapter 6

DOUBLE INDEMNITY: SUBSTANCE USE AND AIDS

Ted Knapp-Duncan and Grant Knapp-Duncan

The use of mood-altering substances has expanded in the U.S. population in the last 25 years to the point that it is estimated that the disease of chemical dependency is a struggle for 10% of heterosexual adults (ages 17–75) and for one third of gay and lesbian people (Finnegan & McNally, 1987). These 25 million citizens combine with 5 million intravenous drug users (Gregorio & Linden, 1988) to constitute a primary AIDS risk group of 30 million.

According to Centers for Disease Control data (1988, January), at least 48% of people with AIDS had a drug abuse history. Of these, approximately 50% are gay and bisexual men who use intravenous drugs and almost 25% are heterosexual IVDUs. In examining these figures, it is important to recognize that CDC statistics tend to minimize the crucial issue of dual diagnoses. Because people with AIDS are listed in CDC statistics under only one risk category, people who are gay *and* substance abusers or bisexual *and* IVDUs are not accounted for as such, despite the recognition that these combined diagnoses are glaring prevention and treatment realities.

By 1992, the Public Health Service predicts that AIDS will be the number two killer of U.S. citizens after cardiovascular disease. This increase in cases can be altered by effective health-promotion, risk-reduction, and disease-prevention programs. The effectiveness of the major programs will be proportional to the degree of cooperative planning among community AIDS

Supported in part by HHS/NIDA grant R18 DA0489903.

counselors, public health planners, and treatment program staff. This chapter addresses issues unique to counseling people whose use of mood-altering substances puts them and others at higher risk for HIV disease. The chapter begins by examining general characteristics of the substance-using population. It then turns to a profile of the HIV-infected substance user and the recovery process. The chapter continues by discussing ways in which the HIV virus is transmitted within the using population and from the using population to the nonusing population. Finally, the chapter examines counselor interventions, describing both assessment and counseling techniques.

The Substance-Using Population

Although IVDUs constitute the second largest group (after gay/bisexual men) of CDC-defined AIDS cases, when they are coupled with those whose chemical dependencies render them incompetent to practice safe sex behaviors, the aggregation swells to a risk group larger than that of gay/bisexual men. Although it has been documented that HIV prevention behaviors have reduced new HIV seroprevalence to less than 1% in the gay/ bisexual community (Winkelstein et al., 1988), chemically dependent IV drug users are still at risk. The AIDS risk-reduction message has not reached drug users with the same impact as it has reached gay and bisexual men. Many counselors and epidemiologists consider substance users to be the "second wave" of the AIDS epidemic.

The substance-abusing population forms a less solidified community than the gay community and thus is less easily accessed for education and prevention purposes. Substance-abusing subcultures do exist. These subcultures often depend on the drug of choice; methamphetamine users, alcoholics, crack smokers, heroin shooters, and cocaine sniffers each may have their own "culture." In areas where many users live, work, and play—for example, urban settings—there will be hierarchies and divisions among users; where there are fewer overall users, there may be more of a passing congregation based on getting high regardless of the substance used. Counselors may find it helpful to view drug using as a behavior that occurs within a particular drug-using culture, rather than viewing drug use simply as a matter of individual pathology.

Drug-using behaviors that put users and their sexual partners at risk for HIV can be understood through the help of ethnography, a science that studies the cultural context (Feldman & Biernacki, 1988). From ethnographic observations, one sees structured sets of roles, values, and status allocations in a previously described "difficult-to-access" population. Rather than being viewed as different, as objects of scorn, fear, hostility, mistrust, and pity, the drug-using population might be considered to be people who do not follow societal expectations as defined by current public policy. Securing and using drugs constitutes a game played between drug users and representatives of the social control system such as the police and the legal system.

The substance-using population, especially IVDUs, tend to distrust much of what they hear, particularly from authority figures. Communication barriers can exist because of ethnic, cultural, and educational differences. Health educators often speak in coded, jargon-laden phrases that sound foreign to substance users at risk for HIV disease, many of whom have low self-esteem and are not motivated to try to understand or remember the message.

Access to health care is a major issue for this population. Substance abusers tend to have an irregular employment history, resulting in a lack of health insurance. If users who are HIV-seropositive do have insurance, they are hesitant to use it for drug treatment program coverage for fear that their confidentiality will be breached or the policy will be canceled. If an individual (regardless of "use status") is between 18 and 55 years old, he or she has a 25% chance of having only Medicaid coverage, which provides minimal services.

Many members of the drug-using population first identify as marginalized citizens dealing with the social legacies of classism, sexism, racism, and homophobia. Compared to the lack of decent and affordable housing, high infant mortality rates, limited educational opportunity, limited job training, institutionalized discrimination, easy availability of handguns, and high teenage pregnancy rates, the threat of AIDS, with its 11-year incubation period, does not seem to warrant much concern.

Other users do not consider themselves marginalized citizens; they are often called "white collar" drug users. College students tested for HIV disease are reported to have approximately half the seroprevalence rate of those in the prison system. This suggests that education and money do not motivate white collar drug users to use condoms more, to share needles less, or to seek treatment more frequently. Instead, these users may be more skilled in denial, bargaining, and intellectualization. Although their manipulative behaviors and verbalizations may be more difficult for health care professionals to deal with, white collar drug users are often able to look at their chemical dependency and increased risk for AIDS. Baum (1985) and Sorenson and Bernal (1987) offered ways in which counselors can encourage their clients to examine drug use patterns.

HIV-Infected Substance Users
and the Recovery Process

The statistics of reported AIDS cases reveal that of the almost 20% of heterosexual IVDUs, 78% are men and 22% are women; Blacks compose 50% of this group, Hispanics/Latinos about 30%, and Whites about 20%. Blacks and Latinos continue to be overrepresented among IVDUs with AIDS as compared to IVDUs in general. These statistics come predominantly from New York, Connecticut, and northern New Jersey where three quarters of all IVDU-AIDS cases originate (Des Jarlais & Friedman, 1988). However, in those states, Whites constitute a smaller proportion of IVDUs than in the remainder of the country.

Of those people who have been diagnosed with HIV disease since the beginning of the epidemic, one half are dead. The others survive with the realities of harboring a chronic, usually fatal virus. If the infected person is a substance user or IVDU, he or she will probably interact with the AIDS health care delivery system or the substance abuse treatment system. Often this involves seeking access to limited resources and facilities. As a result, many continue to live in denial of their substance abuse and without knowledge of their HIV serostatus. Some lower income seropositive IVDUs attempt to "spend down," exhausting what little financial resources they have in order to qualify for public health services. Others continue life on the streets or find temporary housing in the limited shelters for the homeless, which often lack proper medical treatment.

Recovery

The user who is HIV-positive and has had knowledge of his or her serostatus for several months may express a readiness for recovery from his or her addiction in the hope of receiving better health care. The concept of "kairos," a potential turning point or opportune and decisive moment, is often used to refer to this expectant and fragile time. Early indicators in persons about to stop using drugs or about to enter a treatment program have been identified. The authors' experiences and those of Biernacki (1987) point to a number of categories of presenting issues that people often express at the beginning of the recovery process. Knowing these "pathways from addiction" may be helpful to counselors working with HIV-infected substance users.

A first pathway from addiction involves the users' "hitting bottom," or acknowledging that there is too much pain in their life. A "bottom" with IV users could be collapsed veins, or a significant accident such as an overdose. Other users may experience intolerable self-blame or feel overwhelmed by their HIV infection. Although bottoms are of all types, most can be framed as decreases in coping mechanisms.

A second pathway may be initiated when a significant other leaves. This could take the form of the death of a partner from AIDS, a loss due to incarceration, or the end of an emotionally supportive relationship. Sexual dysfunction may become pronounced or sexual phobia may enter the relationship as a result of the partner being HIV-seropositive. The "significant other" could be the user's drug-using friends (his or her "running buddy" or "copping partner"), or even the drugs themselves. The loss might result from the user's drug supplier becoming sick or getting arrested. This large category acknowledges the interaction and interdependence (even codependence) of the user and others in his or her social networks.

A third pathway occurs when users seem to mature out of their habits; they recognize that they are aging. Particularly in HIV-infected users, there may be an extremely disturbing decline in general physical health and appearance. Other users may simply desire more stability in their lives as they reach 30 or 40 years of age. Recent work with female users suggests that women may be more responsive to maturation effects than men (Murphy, 1987; Murphy, personal communication, 1988).

A fourth pathway involves a personal existential crisis, common in the face of the AIDS epidemic. Occasionally a significant visionary or conversion experience is reported. Suicide attempts and some overdoses fall into this category. Increased religiosity or even moral self-ostracism from the using population can put the user into kairos. Being hospitalized for an opportunistic infection may offer the user a more contemplative environment that could foster an idiosyncratic and self-identified crisis and result in a desire for drug recovery.

The Spread of AIDS

The spread of AIDS in the substance-abusing population occurs via two primary vectors. Substance abusers transmit the HIV virus to other abusers through the use of blood-contaminated needles. In addition, as with other populations at risk for AIDS, substance users spread the HIV to other drug users and nonusers alike through unsafe sexual practices.

Spreading AIDS Through Unprotected Sexual Practices

As with other populations at risk, AIDS in substance users is spread through unsafe sexual practices. In 1988, Feldman, Biernacki, and Knapp-Duncan conducted extensive interviews with 295 IVDUs in San Francisco who were identified through chain referral and targeted sampling (Watters & Biernacki, in press). Of this group, 70% of the drug users believed that AIDS can be transmitted sexually to and from partners. However, despite their knowledge, only 42% acknowledged using condoms or other types of latex protection. This figure is alarming in light of the fact that 81% of these IV drug users reported having had sex with at least one person in the preceding 6 months. Although the HIV status of this specific group of IVDUs was not specifically known, blood testing of overlapping samples in the same neighborhoods yielded a 15% seroprevalence rate (Watters, 1987).

Substance abusers who do not shoot drugs intravenously are *not* free from the risks for AIDS. The primary risk to these non-needle-using substance users is from disinhibition because of their substance-induced "high." The euphoric and disinhibited feeling during alcohol or drug use affects the user's judgment, "allowing" the user to engage in high-risk sexual acts despite the knowledge of AIDS risks.

Corollary AIDS risks to non-needle drug users are the immunosuppressive effects of alcohol, cocaine (crack and powder), amphetamines, marijuana, and other hallucinogens (Siegal, 1986). Steady substance users exhibit decreased resistance to infection, substandard nutritional status, and increased susceptibility to common environmental viruses. Many users have experienced health problems including pneumonia, hepatitis, endocarditis, tuberculosis, and cirrhosis (Allen & Curran, 1988). Their immune systems may be in a chronic state of suppression, thus offering the HIV a receptive host. The opposite of this may also hold true; Scott (1988) has found that recovery from substance abuse seems to have an impact on slowing the progression of HIV.

In considering sexually transmitted AIDS in substance abusers it is important to remember that the users themselves are not the only ones affected. Sexual partners of drug users and their children are also at risk for AIDS. Perinatal transmission issues are common among female drug users and the female sexual partners of users. Perinatal transmission occurs 50% of the time between an HIV-positive mother and her child. Disease prevention measures such as nonpenetrative sex or the use of nonoxynol-9 lubricants with latex protection (condoms/rubber dams) would prevent this transmission; however, substance users (both men and women) and their partners must have knowledge of and access to these prevention measures before they will employ them. Counselors engaged in education with substance-using populations must be well-versed in the multiplicity of issues surrounding women's issues and HIV transmission (Mays & Cochran, 1988). Care must be taken when discussing safer sex practices that are also birth control measures, especially among cultures sensitive to imposed genocidal practices (e.g., forced sterilizations or abortions), and among cultures where spiritual beliefs do not embrace family size limits. The counselor should not hesitate to make a referral to outside agencies that can provide additional education about these sensitive issues, thereby ensuring that the client has the best information and care available.

Spreading AIDS Through Blood and Needles

The prominent risk in this second category of the spread of AIDS is through the use of IV drugs without cleaning needles and "rigs" or "works" between uses and users. Needle hygiene among IVDUs is reported to be used only 75% of the time after 2 years of an innovative, street-based outreach program (Feldman & Biernacki, 1986, 1988; Watters et al., 1988). Needle hygiene behaviors among IVDUs in cities other than San Francisco are much less frequent (e.g., Des Jarlais, Casriel, & Friedman, 1988; Becker & Joseph, 1988).

The previously discussed Feldman, Biernacki, and Knapp-Duncan study in 1988 found that intravenous drug users were more careful with regard to needle hygiene than to safer sexual practices. Most of the sample of IVDUs (70.2%) reported never reusing "rigs" without cleaning them. These results replicate and extend those of Watters (1987), who reported that needle cleaning among a sample drawn from the San Francisco IVDU population rose from 39% in 1986 to 76% in 1987. In contrast, the use of condoms was reported to have increased only from 23% to 31% during that year (Watters). This suggests the existence of a greater resistance, at least among the IVDUs in San Francisco, to practicing safer sex than to implementing clean needle hygiene. Counselors who are mindful of the above data can structure their clients' risk assessment around unprotected sexual risk (including perinatal) as well as the more direct risk from shared needles.

Assessment

Counselors working with both substance *using* and substance *abusing* clients will want to assess their clients for the risk of exposure to the HIV. In addition, counselors will want to take an inventory of how receptive these clients are to implementing of the behavioral changes that AIDS prevention methods demand. Counselors will need to assess the amount of information about AIDS and the transmission of the HIV that clients have. They will also need to be aware of any limits to the amount of new information clients are able to incorporate into their lives. Counseling clients with a high probability of risk for AIDS is most effective when it is built on some type of plan that incorporates client history. Clients' risk levels must be assessed near the outset of treatment either by semistructured interviewing or by an instrument such as AIDSRISK (Polaris Research & Development, 1988).

The AIDSRISK instrument has three components: a quantifiable risk assessment questionnaire, a counselor case record and counseling issues planning guide, and an extensive, 200-plus page counselor manual. This manual provides detailed guidance for counselors in the planning and delivery of risk reduction counseling. AIDSRISK is appropriate for people of all ages, for gays and lesbians, and non-gays and non-lesbians alike. The instrument has separate scales for men and women. The risk assessment results from AIDSRISK are compiled in an easy-to-understand "thermometer" that visually communicates the estimated level of risk.

Counselors using a nonstructured assessment interview should include questions related to past risk behaviors such as unprotected sexual activities, intravenous drug use, "recreational" or other drug use, and use of blood products, including transfusions; it is best to get a 15-year history. It will be useful for counselors to be sensitive to a client's family history of substance use and abuse, and any evidence of sexual abuse. Although each counselor's clinical judgment should guide the inquiry and his or her personal style should dictate its framing, the authors advocate an informal, but not client-centered, approach with drug-using clients.

Counselors will also want to assess their clients' openness to the changes necessary to implement safer sexual practices. In large part, the drug- and alcohol-using community operates around short-term goals, not long-term disease prevention plans. Clients' attitudes toward nicotine, smoking, and lung cancer might be explored as a means of assessing their capacity to understand and incorporate long-term changes. Similarly, counselors can explore clients' attitudes toward caffeine, dietary salt, or sugar as a general indicator of the clients' health consciousness. If the using client can understand, through the assessment sessions, the value of longer term health goals, then major behavioral changes may be possible. If clients' immediacies or basic needs are paramount, then perhaps the biggest gift a counselor can give them is to expand his or her professional role to that of a superbly knowledgeable referral source (Kagle, 1987) and to keep clients coming back—or go to them.

Assessment also needs to be made of the client's knowledge of HIV and its transmission. Although much of this may already have been addressed during history-taking, any areas that were not covered should be focused and elaborated on, especially facts about HIV a particular client needs to hear. This assessment might include the discussion of topics such as the pros and cons of HIV antibody testing, confidential testing versus anonymous testing, and the value of testing as a part of an overall strategy for health promotion, risk reduction, and disease prevention.

Often the counselor is tempted to impart far more information than the client is willing or able to incorporate into his or her life. This kind of overeducating through talk may relieve the counselor's anxieties, but may not be appropriate for the client. Many clients may not be psychologically capable of directly dealing with even factual information about AIDS at initial sessions with counselors; pamphlets are often helpful for later reading. Counselors need to remember that information about AIDS is not a sufficient intervention. Tools for behavior change are critical components of an effective strategy. These tools include no-cost detox or treatment programs, bleach in easily usable containers, and needle exchange programs (Des Jarlais & Friedman, 1988).

Implications for Counselors

Successful AIDS counseling programs for substance abusers have four basic components. Cognitive, attitudinal, behavioral, and environmental factors are all integral parts of AIDS prevention with drug users. Table 1 delineates a variety of specific issues that influence AIDS prevention efforts with IVDUs. These components and factors must be incorporated in counselor education programs in order to be effective.

Cognitive components of successful counseling programs for substance abusers address the amount of knowledge they have about different AIDS-related issues. Education geared toward cognitive change must instruct substance abusers on AIDS transmission, needle hygiene, and safer sex practices. Counselors must also provide substance users with locations, directions, and phone numbers for local drug treatment centers as well as health and social service agencies.

Attitudinal components of successful counseling programs for substance abusers examine the beliefs, attitudes, and values substance abusers hold that may prevent them from stopping the spread of AIDS. Counselors will need to address factors that motivate clients to adopt a healthy life style. Counselors

TABLE 1

Components of Successful AIDS Prevention, Education, and Counseling With Substance Abusers

Cognitive

Knowledge of AIDS and its means of transmission
Knowledge of needle hygiene
Knowledge of safer sex practices
Knowledge of drug treatment and other local health and
   social service resources

Attitudinal

Motivation to maintain/promote health
Beliefs about riskiness of one's practices
Attitudes about self-efficacy
Values about sex, sexual practices, and procreation
Self-esteem
Esteem for peers as models/educators
Attitudes about health and human services agencies

Behavioral

Drug user profile
Needle-sharing/hygiene practices
Sexual practices
Language and literacy
Basic life skills
Use patterns of health and human services, including
   drug treatment
Residency
Job skills and employment history

Environmental

Drug use patterns
Hangouts
Systematic connections between substance-using groups
Law enforcement practices
Availability of housing and employment opportunities
Access to health and human services agencies
Access to AIDS service organizations
Access to community-based organizations

will need to review clients' beliefs about the riskiness of sexual practices. At the same time, clients' values about sex, sexual practices, and procreation must be taken into consideration. Clients' self-esteem and their perception of self-efficacy are also attitudinal considerations of successful counseling programs.

Finally, how a substance user views peer educators and health and human service agencies needs to be addressed.

Behavioral components of effective counseling programs with substance users focus on eliciting changes in risky and unhealthy behaviors. Needle sharing, needle hygiene, sexual practices, and basic life skills are target areas for behaviorally oriented counseling. Enhancing clients' job skills and helping clients find housing also fall under this category.

Environmental components of successful AIDS counseling programs for substance users take into account the influences that various patterns, locations, and cultural factors exert on substance users. Counselors will need to address ways that recovering substance users can break away from old hangouts, old drug-using friends, and old illegal activities or patterns. On a broader scale, environmental components of successful counseling programs involve making resources available to HIV-infected substance users. Counselors need to become active in legislation and other activities that will help establish health and human service agencies, AIDS service organizations, and community-based organizations equipped to handle the special issues of HIV-infected substance abusers.

Many clients may initially approach counselors seeking only accurate information on AIDS. As counseling progresses, other issues may arise such as death and dying, spirituality, coming out, and recovery. AIDS issues are often a client's presenting concerns that seem to touch all areas of his or her life.

Whether counselors serve in institutional settings, familial settings, in clerical or pastoral settings, or in a "street" setting, their most effective tool will be a nonjudgmental attitude. AIDS counseling with substance abusers demands that counselors drop their professional veneer; it encourages counselors to be neighborly and natural and to be more personally open than usual. Regardless of what counselors see and hear of marginally legal or even illegal drug activity, they must make AIDS prevention their primary focus.

As mentioned in Table 1, counselors need to incorporate culture-specific values, norms, attitudes, and expectations to produce useful services (Peterson & Marin, 1988). The using population varies by ethnic group, by sexual orientation, and by neighborhood norms. Counselors will talk with members of conventional and, more often, unconventional families of substance users.

It will be helpful for counselors to identify in some way with the substance abusing population. One way counselors can facilitate their own identification with substance abusing clients is to go through the process of self-inquiry. Counselors can examine their own position in today's success-driven, upwardly-mobile, more-is-better, avaricious society. Counselors can recall their own failures, their own personal "bottoms." Counselors can remember what it felt like when they had no trusted social support system. Counselors will grow professionally and personally by confronting these issues as they work with substance using populations (McKusick, 1988).

Conclusion

Substance users compose a population severely affected by AIDS. Substance users contract AIDS through two primary routes of HIV transmission: the use of unclean intravenous needles or other blood-contaminated drug apparatus and unsafe sexual practices. Substance abusers who are also HIV-infected must contend with dual stigmatization. Counselors working with such clients will have to attend to both recovery issues and AIDS-related issues. In light of the prevalence of HIV infection in the substance-using population, counselors will want to undertake some type of AIDS assessment with most of their drug- and alcohol-abusing clients. Counselors will need to be conscious of cognitive, attitudinal, behavioral, and environmental factors unique to the substance-using population as they engage in the valuable task of helping clients confront the problems of substance abuse and AIDS.

References

Allen, J.R., & Curran, J.W. (1988). Prevention of AIDS and HIV infection: Needs and priorities for epidemiological research. *American Journal of Public Health, 78*, 381–386.

Baum, J. (1985). *One step over the line: A no-nonsense guide to recognizing and treating cocaine dependency*. San Francisco: Harper & Row.

Becker, M.H., & Joseph, J.G. (1988). AIDS and behavioral change to reduce risk: A review. *American Journal of Public Health, 78*(4), 394–410.

Biernacki, P. (1987). *Pathways from heroin addiction: Recovery without treatment.* Philadelphia: Temple University Press.

Des Jarlais, D.C., Casriel, C., & Friedman, S. (1988). The new death among I.V. drug users. In I.B. Coorless & M. Pittman-Lindeman (Eds.), *AIDS: Principles, practices, and politics.* (pp. 135–150). Washington: Hemisphere.

Des Jarlais, D.C., & Friedman, S. (1988). The psychology of preventing AIDS among intravenous drug users. *American Psychologist, 43*(11), 865–870.

Feldman, H.W., & Biernacki, P. (1986). *The empirical basis for preventing the spread of AIDS among intravenous drug users in San Francisco.* Paper presented to the 15th International Institute on the Prevention and Treatment of Drug Dependence. Amsterdam, The Netherlands.

Feldman, H.W., & Biernacki, P. (1988). The ethnography of needle sharing among intravenous drug users and implications for public policies and intervention strategies. In R.J. Battjes & R.W. Rickens (Eds.), *Needle sharing among intravenous drug abusers: National and international perspectives* (pp. 28–39). NIDA Research Monograph No. 80.

Finnegan, D.G., & McNally, E.B. (1987). *Dual identity: Counseling chemically dependent gay men and lesbians.* Center City, MN: Hazelden.

Gregorio, D.I., & Linden, J.V. (1988). Screening prospective blood donors for AIDS risk factors: Will sufficient donors be found? *American Journal of Public Health, 78*(11), 1468–1471.

Kagle, J.D. (1987). Secondary prevention of substance abuse. *Social Work, 32,* 446–448.

Mays, V.M., & Cochran, S.D. (1988). Issues in the perception of AIDS risk and risk reduction activities by Black and Hispanic/Latino women. *American Psychologist, 43*(11), 949–957.

McKusick, L. (1988). The impact of AIDS on the practitioner and client: Notes for the therapeutic relationship. *American Psychologist, 43*(11), 935–940.

Murphy, S. (1987). AIDS and the social sciences: Review of useful knowledge and research needs. *Reviews of Infectious Diseases, 9*(5), 980–986.

Peterson, J.L., & Marin, G. (1988). Issues in the prevention of AIDS among Black and Hispanic men. *American Psychologist, 43*(11), 871–877.

Polaris Research & Development. (1988). *AIDSRISK.* San Francisco: CAPE Publishing.

Scott, N. (1988). Is AIDS always fatal? Siegal says "No!" *Alcoholism and Addiction, 8*(5), 14–16.

Siegal, L. (1986). AIDS: Relationships to alcohol and other drugs. *Journal of Substance Abuse and Treatment, 3,* 271–274.

Sorenson, J.L., & Bernal, G. (1987). *A family like yours.* San Francisco: Harper & Row.

Watters, J.K. (1987). *AIDS preventing human immunodeficiency virus contagion among intravenous drug users: The impact of street-based education on risk-behavior.* Paper presented to the III International Conference on AIDS, Washington, DC.

Watters, J.K., & Biernacki, P. (in press). Targeted sampling of hidden populations: An emerging research methodology.

Watters, J.K., Case, P., Huang, K.H.C., Cheng, Y.T., Lorvick, J., & Carlson, J. (1988). *HIV seroepidemiology and behavior change in intravenous drug users: Progress report on the effectiveness of street-based prevention.* Paper presented to the IV International Conference on AIDS, Stockholm, Sweden.

Winkelstein, W., Wiley, J.A., Padian, N.S., Samuel, M., Shiboski, S., Ascher, M.S., & Levy, J.A. (1988). The San Francisco Men's Health Study: Continued decline in HIV seroconversion rates among homosexual/bisexual men. *American Journal of Public Health, 78*(11), 72–74.

Chapter 7

CULTURALLY SENSITIVE AIDS COUNSELING

Sally Jue and Craig D. Kain

Many consider acquired immune deficiency syndrome (AIDS) to be a White gay male disease. This view is reflected in the portrait of the "typical" person with AIDS in the AIDS education and prevention materials written primarily in English, and in the lack of culturally sensitive health and social service agencies specializing in AIDS. This stands in stark contrast to the facts: There is a disproportionate percentage of AIDS cases among Blacks and Hispanics compared to their percentages in the general population (Heyward & Curran, 1988).

Mays (1988) suggested that before AIDS prevention efforts can be truly effective it is important for counselors to know the issues intimately associated with everyday-life realities of overlooked or misunderstood populations; the same holds true for effective counseling. This chapter examines AIDS issues from a culturally sensitive perspective—a perspective that honors and respects the diversity of all clients regardless of ethnicity, minority standing in society, or lowered socioeconomic level. After considering general issues in culturally sensitive counseling, issues for minority clients at risk for AIDS are presented.

The Culturally Sensitive Counselor

Culture can be defined as attitudes, values, and beliefs that influence self-perception, self-expression, and perceptions of others. Whether born in this country or elsewhere, ethnic minority people retain, in varying degrees, aspects of their culture and language. In addition to differences between minority cultures and the majority culture, differences exist within each minority group. For example, Hispanics come from many countries in Central and South America and the Caribbean in addition to those born here. Asians, both those born in the United States and those who have immigrated, represent over 100 languages and dialects from nearly 40 countries and territories. Black Americans who are raised in the urban North differ from Blacks raised in the rural South and those who have emigrated from the West Indies and Africa. Each group has diverse ways of expressing themselves, diverse ways of coping with problems, and therefore diverse ways of meeting their needs. Given the diversity both between these groups and among these groups, counseling interventions appropriate for White Americans will often be inappropriate and ineffective.

Often counselors are unaware of how culture influences their interpretations of behavior and thus the outcome of counseling. Often clients, as well, are unaware of these influences. Counselors working with ethnic minority clients with AIDS and their families must have an understanding of their clients' cultural values and how these values influence behavior. An exploration of cultural differences through open discussion can be beneficial to both the client and the counselor. The client, with the counselor's assistance, will need to explore and distinguish between what are cultural issues and what are personal issues. Through understanding and supporting sexual or ethnic differences, the counselor can alleviate confusion, facilitate the breakdown of internalized negative stereotypes in the client, and help raise the client's self-esteem. Providing positive cultural reinforcement for Blacks and Native Americans is especially helpful because American society has a long history of destroying its original culture. For a counselor to support the differences between cultures, he or she must be sensitive to the impact of culture on the counseling process. Counselors, particularly those doing AIDS work, will need to expand their skills and knowledge in order to incorporate concerns raised in at least four areas: stigmatization, traditional cultural healing methods, cultural views of counseling, and the role of the therapist.

How Does a Group Handle Stigmatization?

AIDS is a stigmatized illness. Herek and Glunt (1988) wrote that persons infected with HIV must bear the burden of societal hostility at a time when they are most in need of social support and that "attempts to avoid such hostility may compromise an individual's health" (p. 886). Because in America the disease of AIDS has been socially defined as a disease of marginalized groups, the stigma attached to AIDS as an illness is layered upon preexisting stigma (Herek & Glunt).

To obtain a better understanding of an individual client's response to AIDS, counselors will find it helpful to examine the client's cultural group's history of stigmatization or oppression in the United States. Counselors will have a better understanding of their clients if they are familiar with how a client's cultural group has been affected by the oppression and stigmatization. Of particular interest is how oppression shapes the group response to outsiders and mainstream institutions. People from oppressed groups frequently have difficulty trusting outsiders and institutions, so initial resistance to self-disclosure or seeking outside help may be more a result of group history than avoidance or paranoia. Three case examples illustrate this point.

Chuck was a 38-year-old Native American who looked very Anglo and had an Anglo name. He had listed his ethnicity as White on the agency intake form. Chuck did not let his counselor know he was a Native American until 3 months later. When the counselor asked why, Chuck replied that it was easier to "just pass." He stated that he'd grown up in Oklahoma near an Indian reservation and that past experience had taught him that "people treat you better if they think you're White." Chuck would often hear people say very negative things about Native Americans, not knowing that he was one himself. He had feared the counselor might be like other people and reject him, so he chose initially to keep his ethnicity a secret.

Althea was a 26-year-old Black woman diagnosed with ARC. A former boyfriend was an IV drug user. Althea stated she was very "upset" with him and worried about her own health. When the intake worker told her it might be a few weeks before a counseling slot opened, she became angry and suspicious and accused the intake worker of not really wanting to help her. When the intake worker explained that they had few counseling staff, that it was difficult for *all* their

clients, and that Althea could call the intake worker if
a crisis arose, Althea became calmer and explained that
ealier that day, at the bank, a White teller had pur-
posely first served a White person standing behind her
in line and that Black people are often "put at the end
of the list."

Boht was a 33-year-old gay man from Thailand
diagnosed with AIDS. He was very nervous during his
first appointment and refused to say much about himself, but asked the counselor several questions about
himself and why and how he chose to work with people
with AIDS. Boht was also very concerned about confidentiality and who would have access to records about
him. The counselor answered all his questions openly
and honestly and did not push Boht to talk about himself. As Boht began to trust the counselor, he began
to reveal more about himself. The counselor eventually
discovered that Boht was undocumented. Boht had
heard stories about how undocumented people were
reported to immigration by agencies that had prom-
ised to help them. In these stories, the undocumented
people always ended up being deported. For Boht,
deportation meant certain death because his own country, he said, could not provide any medical treatment
for his oppportunistic infections.

These three cases illustrate how oppression and stigmatization result in minority clients' distrust of counselors and counseling institutions.

What Are the Client's Traditional Healing Methods?

The client's cultural beliefs about illness, death and dying,
and appropriate medical treatment are essential information
for a therapist working with people with AIDS from diverse
cultures. Some clients may prefer their traditional cultural healing arts to Western medicine. Exploration of these issues may
lead to a discussion of the client's spiritual beliefs that may play
a key role in the client's coping methods, suicidal risks, and
decisions about the use of artificial life support systems. The
following two vignettes illustrate the importance of traditional
healing methods to clients.

Bart was a 43-year-old Native American diagnosed with AIDS. He was deteriorating rapidly and had lost faith in conventional medical treatment. Bart wanted to see a Native American medicine man whose tribal culture was closest to his own. He stated that he could not be at peace with himself or die with dignity unless he could undergo a tribal purification ceremony to cleanse his spirit and reconnect it to the earth and all living things.

Rafael was a 47-year-old gay Mexican American who had toxoplasmosis. He lived with his 30-year-old Anglo lover. Rafael was depressed because of his diagnosis though physically he felt fine. Individual therapy and reassurances by his physicians did not alleviate his depression. His family in Mexico had found a curandero, or folk healer, and wanted to pay for the healer to live with Rafael and work on him for a month. Though his lover was skeptical, he agreed, and with the support of his AIDS support group members, Rafael told his family to send the healer. Though the healer's practices were unorthodox by Western medical standards, Rafael's belief and participation in her healing rites did alleviate his depression.

These two vignettes illustrate the key role a client's traditional spiritual beliefs play in the client's process of coping with AIDS.

What Are a Particular Culture's Views of Counseling?

The definition of emotional support varies from culture to culture. Culturally sensitive counselors will need to examine a culture's social and familial roles with their AIDS-infected clients. Whether or not the needs of the individual take precedence over the needs of the group will yield information about where a client may seek support, how and when he or she may request it, and what type of support he or she may find acceptable. Clients from some cultures may view counseling as supportive and a way to lessen the burden on friends and family, whereas others may view setting an appointment to discuss highly personal matters with a stranger as bizarre behavior. The following case illustrates this point.

Calvin was a 32-year-old gay Chinese man diagnosed with AIDS. Because he was unmarried, he lived
with his parents and helped care for them. They did
not know that he was gay or had AIDS. He told them
he had leukemia because he did not want them to feel
ashamed of him. Calvin denied any need for counseling though he often felt depressed stating that "counseling was only for real sick or crazy people." However,
he would often call or visit the counselor to obtain
information and, over time, would begin to discuss
some personal feelings. As long as the relationship
remained unofficial, Calvin considered the counselor
a "friend at the agency" and could therefore receive
supportive therapy without having to take on the stigma
of needing counseling.

This example illustrates the impact a client's culture may
have on his or her view of the counseling process.

How Does a Culture View the Role of the Therapist?

Clients with AIDS are clearly in the vulnerable position of
seeking help. Counselors, therefore, are responsible for making
an effort to get to know the client within the client's cultural
context. Counselors will often have to develop a more personal
relationship with the client. This will help establish trust and
alleviate the client's anxiety about the therapist's willingness and
ability to transcend cultural differences. A more personal relationship may take the form of a counselor being asked about
his or her family, sexual orientation, or motive for doing AIDS
work. Counselors may also find themselves in the position of
accepting small gifts, making home visits, and even sharing a
meal with the client and the client's family. Refusing small gifts
or refreshment during home visits would be a rejection of the
client's attempt to show appreciation. Such a refusal would seriously alter if not end the relationship. The following example
illustrates such a case.

Maria was a 24-year-old Hispanic woman who was
diagnosed with AIDS 6 months after her husband, an
IV drug user, had died of AIDS and 2 months after
her 3-month-old son was diagnosed with AIDS. She
also had two other young children and had recently

moved in with her parents for financial and emotional support. Her parents were supportive but anxious about AIDS transmission. Maria started seeing a counselor shortly after her husband died. Not wanting to over-burden her parents and felling unable to discuss AIDS with her other friends, she was especially grateful for the support counseling provided. When Maria was dis-charged from the hospital after her second episode of pneumocystis and was too ill to come in for her coun-seling appointment, the counselor offered to make a home visit. Maria and her family were very pleased. When the counselor arrived, the whole family greeted her, offered refreshment, and insisted she stay for lunch. When the counselor left, they insisted she take the leftovers and thanked her again for all her help. Maria later confided to the counselor that her sharing a meal with the family alleviated their fears about AIDS being transmitted through food and meal sharing.

This example illustrates the need for counselors to tran-scend cultural differences when doing AIDS work. These cul-tural differences are examined in the next section.

Issues for Minority Clients At Risk for AIDS

Counselors working with clients at risk for AIDS either in a counseling forum or in an educative capacity need to be aware of *specific* issues affecting people from diverse cultures in ad-dition to the more *general* considerations discussed above. Ad-mitting that AIDS affects minority communities also means acknowledging the existence of homosexuality, bisexuality, and the use of intravenous drugs. When people are diagnosed with AIDS, they can no longer easily hide their life style or behavior. They must face the stresses that accompany the conflict of de-termining whether or not to disclose their diagnosis and life style to significant people in their life. In working with minority clients, it is important to examine these issues within the cultural context of each ethnic group. Because the behavior and atti-tudes of those infected with HIV via high-risk sexual behavior differ from those infected with the virus via drug use, and the behavior and attitudes of men differ from those of women, each will be discussed separately. First, it is important to examine the common ground encompassed in how different cultures view AIDS.

Attitudes Toward AIDS

In his book, *A Strange Virus of Unknown Origin*, Leibowitch (1985) refers to "AIDS à l' Américaine." From his French perspective, Leibowitch writes:

> The AIDS film is an international production on the scale of the media network. But the script is American and carries the cultural insignia of its origin. To tell, to make known, to announce the disease and death—to inform the patient of the medical procedures that will follow, to obtain his [sic] informed consent, to expose and to discuss while exposing—North America has its cultural features. The dramatization that results from this relation to discourse, to exposure—what sometimes for us, prudish and evasive Latins, assumes the quality of an obscene voyeurism—has been, from the start, the trade mark of AIDS à l' Américaine. (p. 93)

Asians and Hispanics, too, view AIDS as a Western or American problem. The small number of Asians in the United States and in Asian countries diagnosed as having AIDS reinforces the belief that AIDS is a Western disease brought on by the high-risk behaviors of Americans and other Westerners. The danger in this belief is the accompanying conviction that if one adheres to Asian cultural norms, there is no need to be concerned about AIDS. The even smaller number of reported AIDS cases among Native Americans leads to a similar denial of AIDS as being a problem with which that population needs to concern itself. Although many Hispanics have heard about AIDS, they may have little information other than "it's a sleazy disease" (Jue, 1988). Sexual behavior is not a socially acceptable topic of conversation among most Asians, Hispanics, and Native Americans, and uncomfortable feelings surface when the transmission of AIDS is discussed.

The belief that AIDS originated in Africa and the inclusion by the Centers for Disease Control of Haitians as a separate high-risk group up until 1986 has adversely affected the Black community. Many Blacks feel there is an underlying message that there may be something intrinsic to Blacks that makes them responsible for the origin and spread of the disease. Thus, the Black community struggles with anger, resentment, suspiciousness and even defensiveness about AIDS while trying to care for the 24% of all AIDS cases that are Black (Centers for Disease Control, 1986).

Issues for Minority Gay and Bisexual Men

Because many men are hidden in their communities where extremely strong taboos against homosexuality exist, there is little information on Asian, Hispanic, Native American, or Black gays and bisexuals. Most of these ethnic cultures consider homosexuals to be men trying to be women or men engaging in isolated sexual behaviors that they can chose to do or not to do. Homosexuality is often viewed as perverted and obscene, a disease to be cured, or a sin against God and nature. Nearly all minority clients voice feelings of isolation. The absence of a supportive environment and the low visibility of minority gay people has helped perpetuate the perception that homosexuality is a White American phenomenon. Gay organizations in minority communities are rare, and those attending to people with AIDS even rarer, leaving minority gays to join the White gay community or remain isolated in their own community.

Because of the oppression of homosexuals in ethnic cultures, many men may engage in same-sex behavior and may choose to continue to define themselves as heterosexual. Peterson and Marin (1988) reported that many authors suggest that men who have sex with other men may not label themselves as homosexual depending upon the meaning of or reasons for the sexual behavior. Men may engage in same-sex behavior for recreational reasons related to physical pleasure, or for economic reasons (i.e., prostitution). They may participate in only "masculine" roles, being the insertor in oral and anal sex. In each of these cases, the man may participate without compromising his self-identified heterosexual orientation.

This lack of a large and viable gay minority community with which to identify and the difficulty minority men have in assuming a personal gay or bisexual identity result in a situation of severe isolation—not only from AIDS care but also from AIDS education. Whereas White gay men receive AIDS education information through gay newspapers, gay bars, and gay organizations, this information will not be available to most ethnic minority gay men. In addition, many of the current AIDS information pamphlets are written in English and at a high school educational level, thereby excluding non-English speaking minorities and those men without higher education. All these factors put minority gay and bisexual men at higher risk.

Of extreme concern to counselors and educators doing prevention and education work are the many erroneous beliefs regarding AIDS some minority gay men hold. One common, incorrect belief is that anal intercourse is safe if one is the active rather than the receptive partner. Another erroneous belief is that high-risk sexual activities are safe if one engages in those activities only with minority rather than with White men (Peterson & Marin, 1988). Part of the acceptance of these erroneous beliefs may be due to lack of education. In a Black community survey in Detroit, Williams (1986) found that Black gay men were less informed about the AIDS epidemic than Black IV drug users, and were unable to correctly identify the modes of transmission of HIV (Peterson & Marin). Peterson and Marin suggested street outreach campaigns employing minority men knowledgeable about AIDS risk reduction and familiar with the sociosexual contexts of ethnic minority communities as a means of combating this isolation and lack of information.

Issues for Minority IV Drug Users

About 85% of all people who contracted AIDS from using intravenous drugs have been from minority groups, primarily Black and Hispanic (Centers for Disease Control, 1986, June 30). Drug users who are poor are more likely than are affluent abusers to share needles or frequent shooting galleries, because needles are difficult to obtain.

Alcohol and nonintravenous drugs contribute indirectly to the spread of AIDS. When one is under the influence of such substances, one's judgment is impaired and the likelihood of engaging in unsafe sex increases. With sexually ambivalent men, drugs may be a way of overcoming inhibitions and later disclaiming responsibility for the behavior. Jue (1987) described a client who stated that he had sex with men only when he was high because he could not handle it any other way. Because of the added stress involved in being gay or bisexual and the prevalence of drugs in some minority communities, minority people are at a greater risk of contracting AIDS from a combination of drug use and sexual behavior.

There is a need to develop appropriate AIDS prevention and education programs in drug treatment clinics in minority communities (Peterson & Marin, 1988). Counselors will need to educate IV drug users about the risks of AIDS either before they are infected or before they infect their partners. Triandis, Marin, Lisansky, and Betancourt (1984) recommended that the programs include ethnic minority staff who would be more accepted by minority addicts because of their knowledge of the minority cultural values, particularly social scripts related to respect and positive social relations. Because IV drug users not in treatment outnumber those in treatment, prevention and education programs are also needed on a "street" level.

Issues for HIV-infected Wives and Sexual Partners

For those men who are more dependent on or emotionally tied to their ethnic community, bisexuality is an alternative to being gay. The fear of exposing their double lives often causes these men to have multiple anonymous sexual encounters outside of their communities. Because these men are most likely to deny the gay or bisexual label or to admit they have had sex with men, their wives have no idea of their extramarital affairs or their risk for AIDS. Many wives may not know about their husbands' same-sex behavior until the devastating time that he or she herself is diagnosed with AIDS.

The wives of bisexual men with AIDS experience anger, betrayal, loss of trust, and fear for their health and that of their young children who may have been conceived while the father was infectious. They may also feel inadequate and ashamed, considering themselves failures as wives and as female sexual partners. Under normal circumstances these women would turn to their families and friends for support. The stigma attached to AIDS and their own sense of shame, whether or not they might also be diagnosed with AIDS, leaves them isolated. The women shoulder the burden of keeping the truth to themselves in addition to caring for their spouses and families with little or no support. This is particularly true if the woman is monolingual. The tragedy is compounded if the woman herself is also diagnosed with AIDS.

IV drug use among minority men indirectly accounts for a large number of minority female cases of AIDS as a result of sexual contact. Female partners of IV drug users are likely to be part of a secondary epidemic of heterosexually transmitted AIDS cases, especially among Blacks and Hispanics (Peterson & Marin, 1988). Many sexual partners of IV drug users may not realize that they are at risk for HIV infection because IV drug users do not usually disclose their serostatus to their partners out of a fear of rejection and lack of emotional support.

A significant problem for minority women is the lack of information not only about AIDS but about birth control as well. For traditional Hispanic, or Latino women in particular, cultural pressures swing toward female naiveté (Mays & Cochran, 1988); this also holds true for Asian Pacific and Native American women. Because being prepared means that one has considered having sexual relations, which is something only "bad" girls do, those women who have access to birth control devices do not always use them.

AIDS education and prevention programs often advocate that women discuss sexual practices and condom use with their sexual partners. This suggestion fails to take into account cultural norms concerning sexual behavior. Mays and Cochran (1988) reported that although AIDS risk reduction messages advocate female initiation of condom use, among traditional Latin cultures authorization for use of contraceptives lies with the husband. They also describe a small subset of Black and Latino women who experience physical and verbal abuse in response to requests that their partners use condoms. In addition, some Black women, particularly those at higher risk for AIDS, have yet to incorporate effective birth control methods into their sexual behavior repertoires in the first place (Mays & Cochran). In many Asian Pacific cultures, condoms are associated with prostitution, so condom use with a spouse or non-prostitute would be an insulting gesture. Peterson and Marin (1988) also mentioned a woman's emotional or economic dependence on a male partner as prohibitive to the adoption of safer sex practices.

Cultural issues also play a role in a woman's decision-making process if she does become pregnant. Many minority women do not believe in abortion for cultural or religious reasons. Thus, if they become pregnant, minority women with AIDS are likely to give birth to children who will eventually develop AIDS.

Implications for Counselors

Many obstacles prevent people with AIDS from seeking professional help. These obstacles are magnified when the person with AIDS is from an ethnic minority group. Often minority clients do not know what counselors do or what counseling is and do not think it makes sense to pay someone to listen to them talk about their problems. They are more familiar with the medical model in which physicians prescribe medication for symptoms. Asians and Hispanics, who have a greater tendency to somatize problems than do Blacks, find it especially difficult to differentiate between somatic complaints and the symptoms of AIDS-related infections (Acosta, Yamamoto, & Evans, 1982).

Rather than hearing a description of what counseling is, clients will find it more useful if the counselor explains how he or she can be of assistance. Minority clients prefer a concrete, directive, problem-solving approach with immediate results (McGoldrick, Pearce, & Giordano, 1982). Minority clients' initial needs include information and referral, advocacy, and assistance in obtaining benefits and concrete services rather than discussion of feelings and life history. Following through on concrete tasks will reinforce the clients' perception that the counselor understands their needs and can be helpful. Afterwards, clients will be more receptive to sharing personal feelings.

Because many clients with AIDS believe they cannot go to their families for help, they are forced to seek assistance elsewhere. For many, it is the first time they have had to negotiate systems outside their communities. If they speak little or no English, the task can be overwhelming. The following suggestions reflect only a few of the issues and influences with which a culturally sensitive counselor doing AIDS work must contend.

1. Counselors working with minority clients will need to build trust. Often minority clients are unsure of how well counselors from different ethnic backgrounds will understand them. This is particularly true when they have difficulties expressing themselves in English. Minority clients perceive the White gay community as having the most knowledge about and resources to cope with AIDS, but are unsure if that community will accept and support them.

Jue (1987) interviewed minority AIDS clients at a large metropolitan AIDS service agency. Those clients reported that to build trust they needed to feel that the counselor cared about them as individuals and that the relationship was personal and not strictly business. What White counselors may view as unprofessional self-disclosures or useless chitchat minority clients may view as an important way to develop a personal relationship. This sharing of information equalizes the power differential in the relationship and enables the client to decide whether he or she can trust the counselor to understand his or her different needs. When clients are undocumented residents, trust is even more important because of their fear of deportation to countries in which medical care for AIDS patients is often inadequate or unavailable and the social climate is less accepting.

2. Counselors working with minority clients must assure clients that their work together is confidential. Some minority clients may be living with parents or have parents visiting who may know the diagnosis but not the high-risk behavior involved. During work with the family, it is important for the counselor to clarify with the client what he or she wishes others to know. Minority clients also may want to know about confidentiality and record-keeping policies because of involvement with illicit drugs or because of precarious immigration status.

3. Counselors working with minority clients must maintain consistency between their actions, nonverbal behavior, and what they say to clients. For all minority clients, actions speak louder than words, so following through on promises made and displaying behaviors consistent with opinions counselors have verbalized to clients is paramount to establishing trust.

4. Counselors must be prepared to work with a minority client's family or with client-family concerns. Families play a huge role in the lives of minority clients. Whether or when to tell the family about the AIDS diagnosis and high-risk behaviors is a major issue for clients, complicated by the fact that many minority clients live with their parents and take care of them. Thus, clients are not only afraid of being rejected but are concerned about who will provide for the parents if they are disowned or die. Many clients have relied on their families for support throughout their lives and may not have a reliable alternate support system, so they have more to lose than many other clients if they are rejected. It may take months for clients to decide how to disclose their situation to their families, and the decision is often influenced by the state of their health.

Because it is unacceptable for Asian and Hispanic families to reject an ill child, clients of these groups sometimes decide to tell their families about their diagnosis when they are so ill they can barely care for themselves. Although the families respond by providing care and shelter, they are not always able to provide emotional support. Therefore, when working with families, the counselor may find it helpful to minimize the stigma of AIDS. In addition, in families in which role expectations are a sign of caring, counselors can focus on how well the client and his or her family have fulfilled their obligations in the past and how they can continue to support each other as these roles change.

Whereas Asians tend to immigrate in families, many Hispanics do not. Those with families outside the United States usually do not tell their parents about their diagnosis unless their families already know they are gay. Many of their families cannot afford to visit them, so alternate support systems in the United States are essential. During the end stages of AIDS, most of these clients prefer to go home so they are with their families when they die. At this point, one's life style and diagnosis are irrelevant, and there is no need to seek medical treatment or to fear rejection.

Jue (1987) described several Black clients who felt they would go to their families only as a last resort. Many adult Black clients think they should be responsible for themselves and not have to depend on their parents. For Native Americans with family living on reservations, returning home would not be a viable alternative; health care available on reservations is poor in general, and virtually nonexistent for AIDS-related illnesses. Blacks and Native Americans, because of similar histories of cultural genocide in the United States, have more reason to deny new problems like AIDS that carry a stigma.

5. Counselors working with minority clients should be prepared to use a translator when necessary. With a subject as emotionally charged as AIDS and its associated high-risk behaviors, it is imperative to find a translator who can remain objective, supportive, and culturally sensitive. The translator must maintain strict confidentiality especially if he or she lives in the same ethnic community as the client. It is also important to evaluate the translator's knowledge and feelings about AIDS; someone who is frightened or judgmental will not be able to translate accurately. The use of a younger child as a translator is inappropriate because it both burdens the child and undermines parental authority. The counselor should discuss his or her expectations with the translator before seeing the client

together. A good translator can also be an excellent resource for learning more about a client's culture.

6. Counselors working with minority clients will need to evaluate their clients' level of acculturation. Whenever a counselor works with clients from another culture, it is essential that he or she evaluate their clients' education, socioeconomic level, command of the English language, and level of acculturation. Because family members adapt in different ways and to varying degrees, counselors may need to alter their approach from client to client and from family member to family member. Differences in acculturation often lead to family conflicts, which can become more pronounced when a member is diagnosed as having AIDS. Clients who are rooted in their ethnic community experience feelings of anxiety and a sense of loss when they leave their secure environment to seek help in an unfamiliar culture that may be unsupportive. The culturally sensitive counselor often becomes the cornerstone of an alternate support system for these clients.

7. Counselors will need to modify their preferred treatment modality to allow for cultural differences. Clients cannot be taken out of the context of their ethnic background, community, or sexual life style. A systems and problem-solving approach is effective, as is counseling that is directive, supportive, and short-term. Group work can be effective if members are carefully screened for their level of acculturation, fluency in a common language, and willingness to participate. The group leader should be directive and focused, and set a tone in which members do not feel overly pressured to reveal themselves or fearful of losing face. A more structured educational focus is useful initially because it provides a concrete service and an opportunity for group members to get to know each other in a less threatening manner.

8. Counselors working with minority clients will have to confront formidable countertransference issues. Working with minority clients forces counselors to confront their feelings about AIDS, death and dying, ethnic minority groups, gay and bisexual people, substance abuse, family issues, unwed mothers, abortion, racism, and poverty. Underlying all of these issues are the counselors' basic cultural and individual values. As clients struggle to redefine themselves and their lives post-HIV infection, counselors in a somewhat parallel process are forced to reevaluate how their own cultural and personal biases influence their perception of clients from other cultures. In many cases,

counselors will need to confront their tendency to view those who are different as inferior or undesirable. This may be manifested in many ways: counselors refusing to work with certain clients because they do not want to make the effort to understand, or counselors minimizing the validity and importance of cultural differences or attempting to impose their own cultural values on the client. Other common dilemmas in working with HIV-infected clients are the tendencies for counselors to overidentify with clients because so many are about the same age, and to become overly involved with clients because their needs are so numerous and resources are so limited. Both situations lead rapidly to burnout.

Conclusion

To preserve their cultural integrity and to ensure their survival, minority communities exert strong pressures on their members to conform to group norms. Because high-risk behaviors associated with HIV infection tend to be denigrated by all cultures, most cultures adopt a blame-the-victim attitude toward people with AIDS. The challenge for counselors is to help clients maintain a sense of cultural pride and integrity without taking on the negative cultural judgments attached to their high-risk behaviors.

Another challenge to counselors will be to expand their concept of what therapy is and how it works in order to accommodate clients who are not acquainted with psychotherapy. Counselors need not cast aside their existing expertise as much as integrate concepts from their own and their clients' cultures into a mutually satisfying therapeutic relationship. Once counselors are able to validate cultural differences, they must then seek the values common to all cultures in order to make a meaningful connection to their clients.

Counselors will be further challenged to take more responsibility for developing culturally appropriate interventions and services to minority clients. This is true not only on an individual basis but also on an agency level. Networking and coalition building enable minority and AIDS agencies to share expertise and learn from one other. Working together is more cost-effective and efficient and provides agencies with an opportunity to expand their perspectives and to overcome ethnic divisions and hostilities.

As the AIDS epidemic continues to infect communities already afflicted by prejudice, poverty, and a scarcity of opportunities, it becomes increasingly important for counselors to address the needs of ethnic minority clients. Each counselor must find his or her own way to face the challenges of becoming more culturally sensitive to the issues that confront minority people with AIDS. Counselors and clients alike must be made aware that without knowledge and understanding *anyone* can become HIV-infected. Because the HIV virus does not discriminate, counselors cannot afford to either.

References

Acosta, F., Yamamoto, J., & Evans, L. (1982). *Effective psychotherapy for low income and minority patients*. New York: Plenum Press.

Centers for Disease Control. (1986). Acquired immunodeficiency syndrome (AIDS) among Blacks and Hispanics—United States. *Morbidity and Mortality Weekly Review, 35*, 655–666.

Centers for Disease Control. (1986, June 30). *AIDS weekly surveillance report—United States*. Atlanta, GA: Author.

Herek, G.M., & Glunt, E.K. (1988). An epidemic of stigma: Public reactions to AIDS. *American Psychologist, 43*, 886–891.

Heyward, W.L., & Curran, J.W. (1988). The epidemiology of the AIDS virus. *Scientific American, 4*, 72–81.

Jue, S. (1987). Identifying and meeting the needs of minority clients with AIDS. In M. Fimbreo & C. Leukefeld (Eds.), *Responding to AIDS: Psychosocial initiatives* (pp. 65–79). Maryland: NASW.

Leibowitch, J. (1985). *A strange virus of unknown origin*. New York: Ballentine Books.

Mays, V.M. (1988). Education and prevention—special issues (section introduction). *American Psychologist, 43*, 948.

Mays, V.M., Cochran, S.D. (1988). Issues in the perception of AIDS risk and risk reduction activities by Black and Hispanic/Latino women. *American Psychologist, 43*, 949–957.

McGoldrick, M., Pearce, J., & Giordano, J. (Eds.). (1982). *Ethnicity and family therapy*. New York: Guilford Press.

Peterson, J.L., & Marin, G. (1988). Issues in the prevention of AIDS among Black and Hispanic men. *American Psychologist, 43*, 871–877.

Triandis, H.C., Marin, G., Lisansky, J., & Betancourt, H. (1984). Simpatia as a cultural script of Hispanics. *Journal of Personality and Social Psychology, 47*, 1365–1375.

Williams, L.S. (1986). AIDS risk reduction: A community health education intervention for minority high risk group members. *Health Education Quarterly, 13*, 407–421.

Section Three

THE PHYSICAL, PSYCHOLOGICAL, AND SPIRITUAL ASSAULT

Section Introduction

Daily life for people with AIDS (PWAs) involves the constant asasult to their physical, psychological, and spiritual being. PWAs live in a world where, as one client stated, "committing suicide is redundant." For counselors to work effectively with people with AIDS, they must understand and be able to empathize with the special issues that PWAs face. This section describes some of those issues.

One of the first things that a person with AIDS must confront is a weakening physical condition. As the AIDS crisis continues, it becomes more common for physicians and counselors to observe psychoneurological complications as a result of HIV infection. In fact, neurological symptomatology may be the first clue to HIV infection in a high-risk person. In chapter 8, Boccellari, Kain, and Shore describe the clinical aspects the AIDS dementia complex produced by the HIV's insidious ability to cross the blood-brain barrier.

Counselors who adhere to a systems orientation know that a crisis involving one member of a system quickly affects all other members. This is particularly true of the crises, large and small, brought on by AIDS. In chapter 9, Curtis describes the impact of AIDS on the family system. Curtis defines family in its broadest sense, allowing him to offer counselors suggestions on working with the "second chance" family as well as the nuclear family of someone with AIDS, the PWA's friends and lovers, as well as his or her husband or wife.

One of the decisions that people with AIDS must make is how to spend the last days of their lives. In chapter 10, Murphy and Donovan describe one option that those in the last stages of life continue to desire: hospice care. They believe that because hospice care is managed by an interdisciplinary team, it offers many opportunities for counselors to become involved.

The chapter also examines the bereavement services provided by hospice caregivers to loved ones that complete the continuum of hospice care.

Although AIDS can be seen as a disease that attacks the body, those who have worked with people with AIDS experience it as a "dis-ease" that also attacks the soul. In chapter 11, on spiritual issues, Ogle eloquently shares a perspective on the deepest and most personal struggle that an HIV-infected person can face. Ogle writes that articulating experiences of "exile" and "calling" are important if spiritual people are somehow to make sense of their lives and losses in this time of AIDS. This chapter includes moving work by members of one parish, successfully struggling to counter the tremendously debilitating feelings of powerlessness AIDS encourages.

The wide scope of this third section of *No Longer Immune: A Counselor's Guide to AIDS* reflects the complexity of the AIDS crisis. Counselors working with people with AIDS, their families, and loved ones must be prepared to expand the scope of the work that they do, facing intense, exhausting, and rewarding challenges. As the chapters in this section suggest, AIDS is more than a disease of the body—it is one of the mind, heart, and soul as well.

Chapter 8

CARING FOR PEOPLE WITH AIDS DEMENTIA COMPLEX

Alicia Boccellari, Craig D. Kain, and Michael D. Shore

An aspect of the AIDS crisis of growing importance to counselors is the ability of the AIDS virus to cross the blood-brain barrier, producing an associated dementia. Counselors find it difficult enough to watch what should be young, attractive, successful clients physically waste away with skin lesions, pneumonia, and other opportunistic infections. Much harder is the struggle of watching these same clients lose their mental functioning, their ability to walk, talk, and comprehend, their ability to feed themselves, to wash themselves, and to maintain their independence. Yet, this is the case with many individuals diagnosed with AIDS dementia complex (ADC).

It is currently estimated that 90% of AIDS patients have evidence of the AIDS virus in their brain at the time of their death (Navia, Jordan, & Price, 1986); as many as 25% of people may present with neurological changes before the development of opportunistic infections (Navia & Price, 1987). In August of 1987, in recognition of the extreme frequency with which the AIDS dementia complex (ADC) is clinically observed, the Centers for Disease Control (CDC) changed the inclusion criterion for individuals who would receive an AIDS diagnosis. Until then, presence of an opportunistic infection like pneumocystis or Kaposi's sarcoma was required. As changed, the current criteria now include ADC as a disorder that warrants an AIDS diagnosis. The diagnostic criteria of the CDC include a positive antibody test for HIV; a negative lumbar puncture, and either a negative CT (computer tomography) scan or MRI (Magnetic Resonance Imaging), *or* findings consistent with atrophy. Ad-

153

ditional criteria include "clinical findings of disabling cognitive and/or motor dysfunction interfering with occupation or activities of daily living . . . in the absence of concurrent illness or conditions other than HIV infection that could explain the findings" (CDC, 1987).

Little has been written specifically about caring for the patient with ADC. Although there are some similarities between this issue and caring for patients with Alzheimer's and other dementias, the patient with AIDS is quite different. This chapter examines the complexities of working with clients with ADC. First though, an overview will be presented.

Overview of the AIDS Dementia Complex

AIDS dementia complex tends to start subtly, and progresses in a slow insidious fashion. Early manifestations cluster around a triad of cognitive, behavioral, and motor symptoms (Navia, Jordan, & Price, 1986). Cognitive symptoms are reflected in the patient's presenting complaints of difficulty paying attention, memory problems, and mental slowing. Patients often report that they cannot think as quickly as usual. Behavioral changes include symptoms such as apathy, withdrawal, depression, loss of spontaneity, and occasionally irritability and emotional lability. One uncertainty with this initial stage is that many of the symptoms described may be symptoms of depression and not specifically those of an alteration in brain function. One of the immediate differential diagnoses that counselors need to make is whether the person exhibits the memory and concentration problems of someone with either a reactive or major depression, or ADC. Of course, both depression and ADC can coexist. Also important to note is that occasionally, some people develop an organic psychosis (Boccellari, Dilley, & Shore, 1988); although this may happen in the early stages of ADC, it tends to occur later in the disease process. Early motor symptoms include complaints of bilateral leg weakness, balance problems, and loss of fine motor control. Occasionally the patient develops a hand tremor. Patients may notice a change in the handwriting, with writing slowness and a sense of arduousness in completing tasks.

In the late stages of ADC people become globally demented. They develop impairment in virtually all areas: memory, language-based abilities, and visual-spatial abilities. Often people deteriorate to the point where they lose the ability to care for themselves and are unable to perform routine over-learned tasks such as dressing, bathing, or feeding themselves. Frequently the behavioral changes will include a growing passivity with muteness and a general unresponsiveness to the environment. Personality changes at this stage can be quite dramatic as well. The patient may forget and become confused and not recognize even familiar people. There may also be behavioral change in the form of agitation, restlessness, or disinhibition. Late stage motor changes include general slowing on motor tasks, ataxia, and increased weakness, particularly in the legs. Mobility problems may be so extreme that patients may be bed-ridden at this point.

Not much is really known about how rapidly people progress from early stage to late stage ADC. Individual differences are great, with some people reaching the end stage of the dementia in as quickly as 3 to 4 months (Navia, Jordan, & Price, 1986), with other people tending to progress at a slower rate. Several cofactors have been suggested. For example, IV drug users seem to progress more rapidly with the dementia than do nonusers. It may be that the IV drug users begin with compromised abilities as a product of long-term substance abuse, and are therefore unable to adapt or compensate as they develop HIV-related difficulties. People with a past history of neurological illness, head trauma, or stroke may also deteriorate at a faster rate. Individuals who are quite physically ill with AIDS, for example individuals who have had three or four bouts with pneumocystis, who are quite frail and fatigued in general, are going to deteriorate functionally more quickly too; they are not going to have the endurance or ability to compensate for their problems.

The Neuropsychology Service at San Francisco General Hospital is finding that in early stages of AIDS dementia, people's immediate concentration and attention abilities are relatively intact or suggest only mild abnormalities (Dilley & Boccellari, 1988). If neuropsychological evaluators use the traditional mental status task of asking clients to remember three words and then ask for recall 5 minutes later, clients may be well able to do this task without difficulty. However, if a delayed memory task is administered to the same patient, it is likely that poor performance will be seen. A majority of ADC patients show

specific difficulty with 30-minute delay memory testing even
when their immediate memory performance is intact.

Neurological examinations often reveal gait disturbance,
ataxia, leg weakness, and hyper-reflexia that may be evident
more in the legs than in the upper extremities (Navia, Jordan,
& Price, 1986). In early stages computer tomography (CT) scans
often look unremarkable, although occasionally they will show
cortical atrophy and ventricular enlargement. MRIs (Magnetic
Resonance Imaging technique) seem to be superior to the CT
scan in identifying AIDS dementia apparently because of the
MRI's sensitivity in visualizing white matter changes in the brain.

How does ADC differ from the well-known Alzheimer's
dementia? Specifically, when Navia and his colleagues began
looking at the brains of people who died from AIDS (excluding
from the series people with known focal infections like toxoplasmosis and CNS lymphoma) 90% of these people did show
evidence on brain pathology of the AIDS virus infiltration (Navia, Cho, Petito, & Price, 1986). The identified abnormalities
were found predominantly in the white matter and in subcortical structures of the brain, particularly the basal ganglia
and the thalamus, with relative sparing of the cortical mantle.
These results led them to conclude that the AIDS dementia
might best be characterized as a subcortical dementia. There
seems to be an affinity of the virus for glial cells, the cells in
the brain that provide nurturance and support to the neurons.
In contrast, Alzheimer's dementia seems to assault primarily
the cortical mantle and is thus identified as a cortical dementia.

Subcortical dementia was first alluded to in 1912 by Wilson
as he was describing the disorder that now bears his name,
Wilson's disease. In commenting on a series of patients with
Wilson's disease, he noted the presence of "psychical symptoms"
(Cummings, 1986). He described a propensity for the development of two constellations of personality changes in patients
with this illness. One type was the appearance of depression
and apathy. The second was that of a more organic psychosis
as manifested by hyperactivity and grandiosity, either resembling a manic type of psychosis, or in some cases resembling a
schizophreniform psychosis. He also noted that when compared
to people with senile dementia or what is currently known as
Alzheimer's disease, the person with Wilson's disease did not
seem to have the same language-based problems, language com-
prehension problems, or naming problems. Patients with Wilson's disease developed many different motor problems whereas

the Alzheimer's patient tended not to do so, at least not in the early stages. These differences are important for it would seem that ADC is a subcortical dementia. Given the higher incidence of depression and other personality changes seen in subcortical dementia (including Huntington's chorea and Parkinson's), it is not surprising to find such problems appearing with the ADC patient.

To provide counselors with an expanded clinical picture of ADC, two clinical case vignettes are presented.

Case one: Tom, a 40-year-old White gay man with a master's degree in architecture, was at the time of evaluation working as an architect. He had no previous psychiatric history, no significant history of substance or alcohol abuse, and at the time of evaluation, had had an ARC diagnosis for about 6 months. He was brought into the emergency room by his lover who reported that he had been having increasing memory problems for about 3 months and that he had also developed a bilateral hand tremor and more recently an unsteady gait. He was also reported to be in danger of losing his job because of poor work performance. Work problems were striking in light of the fact that Tom had worked for the same company for over 10 years and had advanced to a high level of responsibility. He was admitted to the neurology service where a neurologic exam proved to be within normal limits except for mild impairment on a finger-to-nose task, and a mildly ataxic gait. A CT scan revealed diffuse atrophy with multiple areas of hypodensity of the white matter felt to be consistent with ADC. Tom was referred to the Neuropsychology Service and administered a battery of neuropsychological tests, which measured a full range of motor, memory, visual-spatial, and abstract reasoning abilities. On a Bender-Gestalt Test (which asks a person to copy basic designs from a sample on a card), Tom distorted the designs by fragmenting them to such a degree that many designs were unrecognizable to the examiner. When asked if the designs looked like the original, the patient replied that they did. Tom suffered from anosognosia, not fully realizing the extent or nature of his problems. Such a condition is common with people with ADC who, early on, complain about some of their problems but as they worsen, they complain less, becoming oblivious. Given Tom's background in architecture, he should have been able to execute these designs flawlessly.

Tom is a generally representative case of ADC. Results from his CT scan were consistent with the ADC diagnosis as well as the presenting signs of motor disturbance. The following vignette presents a different kind of case.

Case Two: Dan, a 35-year-old gay White male accountant with an ARC diagnosis of 1 year was continuing to work at the time he was evaluated. Approximately 2 months prior to being hospitalized, he began having memory problems. His lover noted that he progressively began to spend large sums of money that they did not have. He also began to demonstrate intense behavioral outbursts and was admitted to the hospital after threatening to hurt himself following a minor dispute with his lover. On admission he was described as irritable, emotionally labile, hyperactive, restless, with grandiose thinking, flight of ideas, and tangentiality. He was also noted to have poor insight into his problems. Dan demonstrated a delusional belief that he had found a cure for AIDS, had cured himself of AIDS, and was going to cure other people of AIDS. The results of a lumbar puncture conducted at the hospital revealed slightly increased protein, which is sometimes found in people with AIDS dementia. A CT scan was done and found to be within normal limits. However, an MRI revealed multiple small abnormalities in the white matter of the brain that was consistent with AIDS dementia. Dan was started on a very small dose (2 mg.) of Haldol for treatment of the agitation and the hyperactivity. He quickly developed fairly severe extrapyramidal symptoms, which necessitated discontinuing this medication. This drug sensitivity is reasonably related to the specific subcortical attack brought on by the virus particularly to the basal ganglia area, which probably compounded the action of the Haldol resulting in a lowered threshold for the development of extrapyramidal symptoms.

On referral to the Neuropsychology Service, Dan was administered an IQ test. Past records showed that at one point he had an IQ of 155 (in the top 1% of the population in terms of intellectual functioning). At the time of his hospital evaluation Dan's IQ was 85. One of the other tests administered was the Wechsler Memory Scale. On one part of this test he was shown a drawing for 10 seconds. It was taken away and he was asked to sketch the drawing from memory. The drawing produced was quite perseverative. His immediate memory was quite impaired. When asked 30 minutes later to draw the design he had initially seen, he did not remember sketching it in the first place, denied that he had drawn anything, and so was unable to produce anything at all.

These 2 cases demonstrate the common pattern of deficits that occur in ADC patients: difficulty on memory tasks, particularly on 30-minute delay, visual-abstract reasoning difficulties, motor slowing, cognitive slowing, and difficulty with mental flexibility. In addition, Case 2 represents an organic-manic variant of ADC. It also highlights the importance of considering an organic psychosis in HIV-infected individuals who are presenting with psychiatric symptoms.

Counseling Interventions

The type of intervention a counselor can employ clearly depends on where a particular client is in the course of ADC. Generally, two stages need to be differentiated. The first marks the early to midstage ADC, whereas the second encompasses mid- to late-stage AIDS dementia. During stage one, individuals can actively participate in their own treatment and management and should be encouraged to do so. During the second stage, the individual's ability to participate in his or her own care is compromised. At this point the counselor or other caregiver needs to step in and take on more responsibility for caring for the individual with ADC, making the decisions and plans that are necessary.

As a bit of background, there are generally three approaches, or theories, regarding the care of the individual with brain dysfunction. The first is a theory of "Restitution of Lost

Functions" that leads to the attempt to bring back lost abilities, restoring what can be restored. Although this theory is often used with people with static dysfunction, for example an individual with head trauma, there is little place for it in working with people with ADC. With individuals with a progressively demential illness, like ADC, where the HIV virus is continuing to attack and destroy brain tissue, it is highly unlikely that a counselor could help a client recover lost abilities.

The second model or theory is that of "Adaptation and Compensation." This second approach is more realistic and is used best during the early to middle stages of ADC. The thrust of this approach is essentially to encourage and reinforce the strengths the individual has left. The goal of this approach is to fully include the patient in decision making. This helps to support and reinforce the individual's self-esteem.

The third model, "Environmental Engineering," focuses on structuring the patient's environment to make it less frightening, less confusing, and more understandable. This approach is best used in the middle to end stages of ADC.

Much of the discussion that follows is, in fact, a common-sense, practical approach. Working with the individual with ADC can at times feel overwhelming. It is therefore important not to lose sight of the basic strength of common sense, a good heart, and hard work.

Stage I—Early to Midstage ADC Intervention: The Adaptation and Compensation Model

The preferred intervention for those in early to midstage ADC is the utilization of the Adaptation and Compensation model. One goal of this stage is education, involving both the patient and his or her family members and friends and lovers, on the physical, cognitive, and behavioral changes that occur with the AIDS dementia complex. Caregivers specifically need to be informed of the behavioral changes that will take place. Many caregivers respond to behavioral problems as if the infected person had some control over them, as if the person is acting deliberately, as if there were a volitional component to the behaviors. Counselors will often hear family members tell the person to "just stop it" when, in fact, the patient cannot control some of these behaviors. For example, the distractibility that is often seen in people with ADC may be attributed by the caregiver to anxiety or disinterest or simply the patient's not paying attention. The patient who may seem stubborn in the face of ordinary requests may be actually demonstrating the mental inflexibility seen in this dementia. The patient who seems easily upset or labile or who is difficult to be around may be exhibiting the behavioral changes and loss of impulse control commonly seen in people with ADC. It therefore becomes essential that people caring for the ADC patient recognize that many of these behaviors are not deliberate and that the patient may have little ability to control them. Of course, one of the counselor's tasks is to help the caregivers distinguish between those behaviors the patient does have control over versus those behaviors over which the patient does not have control.

Educating family members and friends can be a difficult task because so much is as yet unknown about this disorder. Although counselors can inform people about certain aspects of ADC, such as what some of the symptoms may be and a little bit of what to expect, it is difficult to answer questions about the course of the illness and how rapidly it progresses because the exact course of ADC has not yet been well defined. In fact, it would seem to have a variable course from person to person. It is important, therefore, in communicating with caregivers, for counselors to respond as honestly as possible and to strike a balance between useful knowledge and the considerable uncertainty that exists.

The education of the person with ADC is often best accomplished within the context of supportive psychotherapy or counseling. This means that counselors need to shift from the traditional nondirective role as therapist to an active role that relies heavily on direct interaction with the patient and the caregiver. Eventually, the counselor may need to function more as a case manager, or as a liaison to other medical professionals, financial advisors, and attorneys.

In addition to individual therapy, it is often extremely helpful to provide couples therapy or group therapy to the patient with ADC and his or her caregivers (family members, lovers, and friends). Group therapy offers the caregivers involved with the ADC patient an opportunity to begin to discuss the role changes that are occurring in the family system or unit. Often the roles change so drastically that a person who was previously the breadwinner, or the person who did most of the cooking or cleaning or paid the bills, is no longer able to do so. With these changes, many times the patient may begin to feel a sense of anger, resentment, and guilt about no longer being able to perform certain tasks. The caregivers may also be feeling some resentment that the person is no longer able to perform his or her previous duties. Caregivers may also feel a sense of despair. These are feelings that people often do not talk about and, when unventilated, can destroy the substance of the relationship. Couples therapy or a group format helps to facilitate the exchange of these types of feelings and information and helps both the patient and caregiver come to a better understanding of how to cope with such changes.

Counselors must also recognize that there are two extreme reactions to the ADC patient that may develop. One extreme is that of denial, whereby both the patient and the caregivers may downplay the seriousness of the emerging symptoms. The patient may be doing this as part of the use of psychological denial or as part of an organic denial where the patient is mentally unable to monitor his or her behavior. Family members may experience intense discomfort in observing the patient's dementia and find it necessary to downplay the severity of the situation. Counselors will hear comments like, "well, he's always been like that; this is nothing new." Typically this stage of denial does not last long, particularly as the dementia progresses and it becomes more difficult for the caregivers to hold onto the stance of denial.

The other extreme may be the tendency for the caregiver to act as if the patient with ADC can no longer do anything independently or successfully. There may be a tendency to take over and take complete charge of what the patient is doing in his or her life. This inevitably leads to problems. One of the main issues that people with terminal illnesses experience is a feeling that they no longer have any control over their life, that they no longer have any power to influence their circumstances. When someone with a terminal illness also develops dementia, this issue becomes compounded by real losses and often the patient feels a sense of complete uselessness and a sense that there is nothing at all he or she can do right. At this stage, it is important that counselors talk to caregivers to identify those activities the patient can still do and responsibilities that can be maintained. This may be facilitated by setting up daily and short-term goals that are realistic and achievable for the patient, and by including the patient in larger decision-making processes at this early stage. The individual should be encouraged to stay active and involved.

In the early to midstage ADC, compensation for cognitive problems can be enhanced through encouraging the individual to keep track of needs and events by writing them down. Often patients will report that they went to see their physician and were given information about their medical status, but by the time they got home they could not remember anything that was discussed. In the course of therapy, it is not uncommon for the patient to be seemingly attentive during the course of a discussion only to telephone the therapist later on during the week saying "I don't remember what we talked about." It may be more helpful in these particular circumstances to bring and use a tape recorder. Thus, when the patient has a need to review conversations, this can be easily done.

It is also important to keep in mind that people with ADC lose cognitive efficiency, so mistakes are common, particularly when going too fast. It is important to give people permission to take their time. Counselors can give this permission directly, and also point out that not everything needs to be done at once. This helps to decrease mistakes that often arise through an impulsive problem-solving style.

At this early stage counselors can reinforce and stimulate general mental activity. Clients can be encouraged to play games like scrabble, card games, or checkers. In moderation these activities are not stressful as much as enjoyable. Such activities are helpful because they reinforce and teach patients something about the manner with which the patient needs to go about paying attention to all activities. A balance needs to be struck, however, between games and activities that are stimulating, challenging, and enjoyable, versus things that are frustrating and mildly difficult.

To be dying from AIDS and to be told one is suffering from dementia is extremely frightening. Everyone has a different idea of what the term "dementia" means. Asking patients and their caregivers to discuss what this term means to each of them helps specifically to address their individual fears. Misconceptions or myths about dementia can then be dispelled and a clearer understanding achieved.

It is particularly important for patients with ADC to avoid fatigue. Fatigue seems to cause a worsening of cognitive problems. Mornings tend to be best, and as the day goes on patients tend to become tired and less able to stay on top of their circumstances. Patients can be encouraged to schedule important appointments at the beginning of the day. Counselors will also want to give people permission to take rest periods during the day, even if it is only a half-hour nap in the afternoon. Counselors also can encourage exercise such as daily walks. Daily walks may help relieve tension and reduce stress and also help keep the patient involved in the world.

Counselors can assist the patient in avoiding stressful situations. For example, a patient with midstage dementia reported going to a government office with his lover to apply for food stamps. While in the overstimulating environment of the food stamp office, with the food stamp worker talking, filling out forms, and phones ringing, the patient found himself getting increasingly irritable and anxious and became confused. He ended up escalating by becoming extremely upset and labile. In talking later to this patient, the counselor was able to help the patient identify the stressful situations in his life. Some situations could still be managed, others required outside assistance. One of the accomplishments that resulted was the sharing of early signs of emotional escalation with the lover, who was then able to move quickly to help out when needed. The patient was told that when he found himself getting irritable, he should not keep it inside, but, rather, tell his lover about it. The lover could then take charge and encourage the patient to take a few minutes away from the situation to help regain composure. Counselors need to recognize that nobody can avoid all stressful situations, and that anticipation, planning, and having alternatives enable a higher level of functioning.

Stage II—Mid- to Late-Stage AIDS Dementia Complex Interventions: Environmental Engineering

As mentioned, AIDS dementia complex is a progressive demential illness. At this time there is no cure for ADC. In the early stages counselors and caregivers can continue to feel a sense of hope. Patients still interact with us, still actively participate in their own care, and still tell us what it is they need. During the mid- to late-stage ADC, life becomes not only a struggle to survive but also a struggle to maintain a sense of one's identity, a sense of who one is in relationship to other people in the world. As this sense of identity begins to erode, persons with ADC may get to the point where they are no longer able to fully appreciate their own needs and are consequently unable to care for themselves. In this second stage, collaboration among counselors, physicians, caregivers, and nursing professionals is essential to successful management. Environmental engineering is often a useful approach for people with mid- to late-stage ADC. People with demential illnesses eventually lose their capacity to be mentally flexible and adapt to changes, resulting in their inability to deal with novel situations. Much of what people do on a day-to-day basis is deal with the complexities of an ever-changing world, and patients with late-stage ADC are incapable of doing this. They may not be able to monitor their own behavior or control their actions.

As patients are unable to change and control their own behavior, the environment has to change for them. Environmental engineering refers to structuring a patient's world to minimize the impact of lost abilities. The more structure that is provided by the environment, the easier it is for demential patients to understand and process the world around them. This is an approach dramatically different from those most people in the helping professions are used to. As therapists and counselors, we generally expect and encourage our patients to change. In this approach, however, health practitioners become instrumental in altering the patient's environment whereby less emphasis is placed on the patient changing. Realizing that the environment can be positively altered gives a new sense of hope, and patients' quality of life can be enhanced. Most counselors and therapists are aware of the importance of keeping people oriented, aware of the time, the date, and geographical location. Our anchors to reality also include knowing who we are, where we are, and a sense why we are there. It is important for the demential individual to be given orienting cues. For example, if the patient is at home or in the hospital, a calendar provides cues to the day, month, and year. Clocks are helpful in keeping people oriented to the time of day; many clients prefer digital clocks to avoid the confusing visual task of distinguishing between the minute and hour hands of a regular clock. In places like hospices or group living situations, current event groups for patients to keep them in touch with what is going on both in the treatment place as well as the rest of the world are helpful. The client's environment should be kept consistent with posted routine schedules. Sudden changes can often cause a worsening of confusion.

It is helpful to keep familiar objects around the patient, particularly if the patient is in the hospital. Caregivers can be encouraged to bring in photographs or personal objects to help the patient feel less afraid. Speaking of familiar names, places, or interests that the patient has had in the past is particularly important. It is also important to keep in mind that for people with ADC, their remote memory may be largely intact. It is best to encourage people to talk about things that they are competent to talk about. When counselors need to quiz patients on what year it is, what time of day is it, and where they are living, it is advisable to follow this with questions that the patient can, in fact, answer. It is best that patients be given only one thing to do at a time. For example the lover of a person with ADC complained to a counselor that he could not get the person to take a bath. In studying this situation, it was realized that for someone who is demential, taking a bath is not the easiest thing because of the many different steps involved. It was not that the patient did not want to take a bath. Rather, he could not organize himself in sequence. Often when a patient refuses to do something, it is helpful to understand the problem by breaking the task down into pieces. Presenting the task one step at a time usually results in increased cooperation. Information should also be presented slowly and one step at a time. Counselors and caregivers should not assume that the person is following what is being said. It is sometimes helpful to have the person repeat back what was said. Although this does not necessarily ensure that the patient *understands* what is being said, it increases the likelihood that the patient at least hears you accurately. If the patient can still read, he or she can be encouraged to keep track of needs and events by writing them down in a diary or daily log.

Counselors and caregivers need to keep in mind that too much or too little stimulation can lead to confusion, agitation, and fearfulness. The patient's living space should be uncluttered. Although friends and family should be encouraged to visit the patient on a regular basis, the number of people visiting at one time should be kept to a minimum.

Conclusions

It is essential to keep all those involved in patient care as fully informed as possible. Yet one element of what we know about ADC has not yet been broached. Often patients with AIDS dementia complex are being cared for by their lovers, who themselves are HIV-infected. It is becoming more common for counselors in metropolitan areas (like San Francisco, Los Angeles, and New York) to see couples where both members are demential. What happens when the caregiver has nothing left to give? What is being done to make sure that both the patient and the caregiver are receiving the kind of services they need? There are no easy answers, only hard questions.

What has been presented to this point has been an overview of the AIDS dementia complex. Representative cases were discussed. Treatment in forms of phase-specific care was described. Last to be emphasized was the importance of recognizing that those who help need help also. Much can be done to improve the quality of life of demential AIDS patients, to prolong their independence, and to foster a continuing sense of personal dignity. Likewise caregivers, family and professionals alike, need to maintain their sense of values and competence in work that is challenging and, at times, draining. This too can be accomplished by focusing on what is possible, working hard, and making a difference. Such is the challenge of AIDS dementia complex.

References

Boccellari, A., Dilley, J.W., & Shore, M.D. (1988). Neuropsychiatric aspects of AIDS Dementia Complex: A report on a clinical series. *NeuroToxicology* 9, 381–390.

Centers for Disease Control. (1987, August). Revision of the CDC surveillance case definition for acquired immunodeficiency syndrome. *Morbidity and Mortality Weekly, 36* (supplement), pp. 3S–15S.

Cummings, J.L. (1986). Subcortical dementia. Neuropsychology, neuropsychiatry and pathophysiology. *British Journal of Psychiatry 149*, 682–697.

Dilley, J., & Boccellari, A. (1988). AIDS dementia complex: Diagnosis and management. *Focus: A Guide to AIDS Research, 3*, 1–3.

Navia, B.A., Cho, E.S., Petito, C.K., & Price, R.W. (1986). The AIDS dementia complex: II. Neuropathology. *Annals of Neurology 19*, 525–534.

Navia, B.A., Jordan, B.D., & Price, R.W. (1986). The AIDS dementia complex: I. Clinical features. *Annals of Neurology 19*, 517–524.

Navia, B.A., & Price, R.W. (1987). The acquired immunodeficiency syndrome dementia complex as the presenting or sole manifestation of human immunodeficiency virus infection. *Archives of Neurology 44*, 65–69.

Chapter 9

TREATING AIDS: A FAMILY THERAPY PERSPECTIVE

John H. Curtis

Little has been written about the family's struggle with acquired immune deficiency syndrome or about the reliance that a person with AIDS, ARC, or HIV seropositive status has on the family. Carter (1986) stated that "the effects of AIDS on the family and friends of the ill, the dying, and the dead and the hysteria surrounding this illness promulgated by many members of the press, and sadly, the scientific community, brings the figure of persons affected by AIDS into the millions." Simon (1988) elaborated on the severity of the effect of AIDS on the family by writing:

> Estimates are that by 1991, there will be 324,000 AIDS cases in the United States. Twenty-one thousand people with AIDS have already died. Taking into account the families, friends, and partners of those with AIDS, the disease will have an immediate impact on the lives of millions of people. Many believe that AIDS is the most serious health problem the United States has ever confronted.

With such an enormous impact on the American family, it is important for family counselors and therapists to explore ways to facilitate a family's functional adaptation to the various dynamics of the diseases associated with HIV. Many of these families will need help in dealing with the realities of the disease. Morin and Batchelor (1984) proposed:

> The mental health aspects of the AIDS crisis affect not only those with AIDS but also the people in their

lives. Lovers, friends, and family are all likely to experience significant distress and may need mental health services. Because AIDS is a mysterious and stigmatized illness, the psychological issues raised for significant others may be more complicated than those for other life-threatening illnesses.

The AIDS crisis presents family counselors and therapists with the opportunity to help families cope effectively. Walker (1988) stated that "surviving with AIDS depends in great part on determination, hopefulness, and improving the quality of one's life." Family-oriented counselors and therapists can help families focus on each of these to the benefit of the person with AIDS (PWA).

This chapter examines the use of a dynamic family approach to working with people with HIV infections and their significant others. After a brief description of family-oriented counseling, the chapter turns to an examination of current research conducted by the author, the results of which emphasize the importance of family involvement in the care of people with AIDS. The chapter continues with a discussion of important family issues, and concludes with implications for counselors.

Family-Oriented Counseling

During the past 30 years, family therapy and counseling emerged as a separate helping profession. Prior to this, the typical mode of therapeutic treatment was based on the interaction of one client with one therapist.

The theoretical development of family therapy has emerged from the concept that the family is a closed system. It is assumed that therapy can best be accomplished when all members of a family living unit are involved. This theory assumes that any change in any member of a family will automatically produce changes in the family system. Therefore, family therapists may see any member of a family separately, but typically prefer to interact with the whole family when dealing with families with AIDS or any other family.

Family systems theorists use a broad definition of the family. "Family" may be defined as the family of orientation, or procreation, or as the voluntary family in which a person receives nurture, love, and care. This latter definition is broader than a blood lineage concept most often used by White middle-class families, and includes the functional concept often associated with rural Black families in which nonrelated persons fulfill kin roles. Prostitutes, homosexual men and women, drug users, and teenagers in gangs often form "voluntary" families where kin terms may be used (sister, brother, mother, etc.) but where there is no blood relationship. For the purposes of this chapter "family" is the group that fulfills the functions of family irrespective of blood lineage.

Although there is consensus concerning the broad definition of "family" by most family systems therapists, there is great diversity in counseling styles. These various styles have been organized into distinct schools of therapy with a variety of advocates for each approach. These schools include the psychoanalytic, behavioral, extended family systems, communications, strategic, and structural family therapies (Nichols, 1984). With the development of family systems theory and the recognition of family therapy as a separate helping profession, treating AIDS patients is an appropriate application of this therapeutic modality.

Research Implications for Family Counselors

Research into the various adaptations to AIDS, ARC, and HIV infection by families in the nonmetropolitan southern Georgia region has been a focus for the present author since 1984. Early studies included a statistical projection of HIV infections (cases of ARC, and AIDS and HIV disease) for each county in the state of Georgia (Curtis & Richardson, 1986). This project was followed by another that estimated probable AIDS-related deaths in Georgia county by county based on the formulas in their earlier work (Richardson & Curtis, 1986).

Preliminary Findings—Research in Progress

Another research project was designed by Curtis and Richardson comparing anticipated responses to an AIDS diagnosis among a homosexual sample and a heterosexual sample. The pilot study began 2 years ago with an in-class survey of 65 southern Georgia freshmen from an introductory sociology class.

They reported, in an open-ended survey, that if they contracted AIDS they would (ranked in order of frequency) :

1. commit suicide;
2. flee the country; or
3. return home to their families for care until death.

The responses suggested that students would want to escape the hardship of AIDS (flight or suicide) if they could. The responses also suggest that more realistically, the students recognized the function of the family in caring for its ill members. This pilot study led to further research concerning what persons think they would do if they were diagnosed with AIDS.

During 1987, approximately 170 subjects were studied by interview and questionnaire to establish their anticipated actions to contracting any form of AIDS. Approximately one third of these subjects were homosexual men studied in a small town gay bar in southern Georgia. The second third of this sample was made up of members of a nationwide gay, lesbian, and bisexual professional group who gave the researchers permission to contact its members by mail. A third group of students from the nonmetropolitan southern Georgia college, who indicated they were heterosexuals, were included as a control group. A preliminary analysis of data in 1988 led the researchers to conclude that after exhausting their financial resources, most subjects from this study, if they contracted AIDS, would probably choose to return to their parents for care until they died.

Although the researchers do not propose that these findings can be generalized beyond the samples studied, the results of both studies suggested that people with AIDS might:

1. terminate their lives so as to relieve suffering and expense for the PWA and his or her family;
2. flee, so as to protect the family from the assumptions they might make if they knew the nature or cause of this disease;
3. exhaust all personal resources so as to remain independent as long as possible; and
4. return home to the family to die.

Regional Differences

Before examining issues for family counselors and therapists, the presence of some major regional variations in the

United States related to AIDS, ARC, and HIV spectrum infection should be explored. In San Francisco on Castro Street on a Friday night one can hear persons openly discussing their HIV-related symptoms and the new experimental drugs they may be trying. In southern Georgia, such a conversation would probably not take place. In general, New York and San Francisco may be a few years ahead of the nation in the number of cases diagnosed and services developed to assist PWAs. Other metropolitan areas probably lag behind New York or San Francisco by 2 years in feeling the full impact of HIV spectrum diseases. Nonmetropolitan areas experience an even greater lag. Consequently, there are vast regions where health care resources are still unprepared to deal with the magnitude of infections projected for this disease. In such regions, the primary education about AIDS is provided by the media, and the typical AIDS health care worker is a minimally trained public health department staff member.

For example, the southern Georgia region has few resources to help HIV-infected persons. Many medical doctors are not sophisticated in their understanding of this disease; until recently a person would often be told he or she had AIDS after a single ELISA test; this is an inappropriate and incorrect use of the ELISA test. A few area doctors admit to being reluctant to treat AIDS patients for fear of becoming stigmatized as the county's AIDS doctor and thereby experiencing a negative effect on their medical practices. In a small southern Georgia community, a transient PWA became ill and went for help to the local emergency room. When the PWA revealed to the doctor that he had been diagnosed with AIDS, the doctor gave him $100.00 from his wallet and urged him to catch the next express bus to Miami, "where they know how to treat this disease."

Wellness Associates, Incorporated, a nonprofit volunteer organization was formed in southern Georgia to provide confidential services to persons with HIV disease, ARC, and AIDS and their family members. All services from Wellness Associates are free. The services most often requested include advice on the AIDS crisis line, referral to medical and social agencies, and a support group for the HIV, ARC, or PWAs. Providing direct services to these persons has yielded numerous case studies that may or may not represent the ways that PWAs, persons with ARC, or HIV-infected persons are treated in other areas. Daily contact with the various clients referred to Wellness Associates and their families suggested the following issues that can be addressed by family counselors and therapists.

Issues for Family Therapists

Family counselors and therapists, people with AIDS, and families must face many issues associated with this disease. The family counselor or therapist views the person with AIDS and his or her "family" as a system. Sometimes family systems will be dysfunctional and family counselors and therapists will want to gear their work toward increasing family members' ability to function in a healthier manner. In other cases, these dysfunctional family systems cannot be made functional. When this happens, the family counselor or therapist can still help family members and PWAs by redefining their goals so as to encourage the family members to cooperate *as much as possible* in the care of the ill (Mohr, 1988). In addition to these therapeutic goals, the following themes will often need to be addressed in family therapy.

People With AIDS and Their Families Often Experience a "Double Leprosy" Effect

People with AIDS, persons with ARC, and people with HIV seropositive status typically come from highly stigmatized groups. In addition to the societal stigma, the seropositive individual may personally feel that he or she is a leper for having any form of HIV infection. Unfortunately, much of society, particularly in nonmetropolitan areas, treat people with AIDS and ARC like outcasts. This results in a "double leprosy" effect with the individual feeling like a leper and the society encouraging that impression. The following case example illustrates the double leprosy effect.

Greg, a 20-year-old gay White man, had tested HIV antibody positive twice. Based only on these tests, a doctor inappropriately diagnosed his as a case of AIDS and transferred him from a general hospital to a small psychiatric hospital where he was treated for depression.

Greg's family history revealed that his father and mother had divorced. Greg and his older brother had been raised by a grandfather, who served as the preacher for a very small, fundamentalist church in a small community. His mother had moved to Texas and remarried. His father remarried a woman with two small children aged 6 and 8 years.

Initial contact with the family was tenuous at best and demonstrated its dysfunctional character. Greg's brother did not want to deal with him because he was a "fag." His father was ashamed of him. His grandfather had publicly stated that he was "going to hell for all eternity." No one showed any interest in Greg. His stepmother announced that Greg could not enter her house because she believed he might pass his disease to her children. The brother's wife was pregnant so they did not want Greg to visit their home. Greg's mother called from Texas to tell him never to visit her and asked that he not let any member of her side of the family know that he had AIDS. Greg's grandparents said he could come live with them when he was released from the hospital, but that he would be restricted to his room. No one was to know that he had AIDS because Grandfather feared he would be fired from his pulpit. In summary, mother, stepmother, and sister-in-law feared the contamination of their children. Father, brother, and grandparents felt they could not cope with the fear of AIDS and its social repercussions in their communities.

Greg's position in the milieu of his community was one of severe stigmatization. When his situation was brought to the attention of a few community leaders, one lawyer suggested that Greg should be "bashed." When the lawyer was asked in a televised interview what that meant, he clarified his response and stated that Greg should be executed. All of this left Greg feeling as though his life were already over.

In addressing the double leprosy effect, family counselors and therapists will need to help infected persons like Greg feel positively about themselves and at the same time help the members of the family to be supportive to their ailing family member. Unlike in many other therapy modalities, the family therapist may symbolically join the family (if it will let him or her do so) and design interventions that will encourage and support family change. Counselors need to pay special attention to the issue of "dual relationships," which are much easier to avoid in metropolitan areas than in nonmetropolitan areas where a face-to-face relationship often exists outside the office.

Families are More Resilient Than They Think

Generally, a counselor must start where the family is and help each member deal with his or her feelings. Learning about a family member's AIDS diagnosis confronts family members with issues related to death and dying as well as issues related to the transmission of the disease. Often the social and sexual behaviors that transmit the disease are judged as immoral.

Family systems counselors and therapists usually propose that families are more resilient than the various members think they are. However, it may take time for family members to accept the fact that one of their members has contracted AIDS. Ultimately, if the family counselor or therapist can keep family members talking to each other about their feelings and interacting with the person with AIDS, many families can learn to be supportive. The following vignette illustrates this.

In December 1988 Don received an HIV-seropositive diagnosis. Because his partner had AIDS, their doctor suggested that Don would also probably develop AIDS; Don therefore chose to tell his parents that he was gay and that he had AIDS. In less than 10 minutes, Don's father and mother packed everything Don owned and removed him from the house. These events left Don devastated and he turned to the local AIDS counseling center where he received great support and a "surrogate" family. With a family counselor, Don worked toward reuniting with his family. Because of a strong southern family tradition of caring for dying members that transcends social prejudice, Don's father made steps toward reestablishing communication with his son.

Family Counselors and Therapists Need To Develop Skills for Working With Gay Couples and Their Families

With the advent of AIDS, homosexual couples are increasingly requesting help with their relationship problems, which are often brought into focus by a diagnosis of HIV disease. Consequently the family therapist must work to overcome any feelings of homophobia or "homo-negativism." Patten (1988) stated, that " . . . therapists, given some education and some positive interaction with gays, can learn to move past their hesitancy and awkwardness in working with people whose sexual orientation they do not share."

Patten (1988) found that gay couples were often angry and depressed after an HIV diagnosis. Fights about how (from whom) they contracted the infection are common. Privately, both might be afraid of losing their partner, of being abandoned. The family therapist will want to help gay couples realize that there is no need to panic. Patten suggested telling fighting ill couples that, "No one is dying right now. Your fighting is just a way of staying close while expressing your fear of being separated." Such reframing is often an effective strategy for the family counselor or therapist.

Family Counselors and Therapists Must Educate Families About AIDS

One of the unique functions of the family therapist is to answer families' questions and to help them pose questions as yet unformulated. Families will need to know that not all PWAs die immediately after a diagnosis. The perceptions of family members living in nonmetropolitan regions are confused, even though there have been public (media) educational programs about AIDS. Many family members do not know enough to distinguish between AIDS, ARC, and HIV disease. They consider "AIDS" as a single disease resulting in instant death.

Families will want to know if there is a danger that they can contract this disease, especially if children can be infected. Family therapists can assure all the members of the family that they cannot contract AIDS through casual contact. Even friends of people with AIDS who themselves are members of high-risk groups share this fear of contagion through casual contact. For example, when gay friends began to visit Greg after his release

from the hospital, many were afraid that they could contract
AIDS from the visit. By watching his counselor treat Greg in a
comfortable and relaxed manner, they became desensitized to
their fear of AIDS. His gay friends soon functioned as his family
during a time when his "blood" family was so uninformed and
afraid of contagion that they could not help him.

Families Need to Adjust to the Person With AIDS's Long-Term Illness and the Probability of His or Her Death

The family therapist may become an agent in the death
education for family members. Many persons are afraid of death
and hence deny its reality. The person with AIDS who has
already been to the hospital two or three times and whose immune system has broken down will need to confront his or her
death. Although family members usually anticipate the death
of an aged member, it is often difficult to plan for or deal with
the idea of the death of the family's younger members.

In *Forum* (1987), Paul Volberding, the director of the AIDS
program at San Francisco General Hospital, stated that the
AIDS health care crisis involves two facets: acute care and chronic
care, with chronic care for AIDS patients posing the most pressing problem and one that will worsen as the number of AIDS
cases increases. Brody (1987) pointed out that the place where
chronic care for the PWA is typically given is in the home. She
explained that caring at home for a person with AIDS, a person
with ARC, or an HIV-infected person may prove to be very
"difficult at best, but is often a labor of love."

Families That are Unable to Provide for a Person With AIDS Require Special Interventions

Many families do not have the funds or the physical strength
to cope with a family member's AIDS diagnosis. In these cases,
counselors and therapists are often called upon to act as advocates and to almost magically provide resources. The following case provides one such example.

Stephen was a young man with AIDS. He was
referred to a counselor by his hospital who called wanting to discuss possible placement for him through a

District Task Force. The hospital administrator had allowed him to stay 2 months after all his medical benefits had lapsed and finally had to insist that Stephen be moved. Because of AIDS dementia complex, Stephen was seldom aware of whether it was day or night and was unable to feed himself. He was totally dependent and bedridden. Stephen's mother was quite elderly and when asked to take him, confessed tearfully that she could not lift him, change him, or give him the care he needed.

Rather than see Stephen left to die on the street, the counselor and task force worked out an intricate plan for Stephen that would guarantee his care. When the administrator of the hospital would no longer provide care for Stephen, an ambulance would take him to his mother's home. The drivers would unload him on a gurney and ring the bell. The mother would refuse him because she could not care for him. The ambulance drivers would refuse to take him back to the hospital and leave him on his mother's porch. The sheriff would watch this transaction and with a staff person from Adult Protective Services [Department of Family and Children's Services (DFCS)] would take custody of this abandoned adult, and call another ambulance to take him to the DFCS office. A judge would be asked to declare Stephen incompetent and abandoned. As an incompetent adult, and ward of the state, there was one hospital in the state where the law required that he be treated.

Cases like Stephen's occur in all parts of the country. As this case illustrates, counselors will need to be familiar with local resources, and the intricate workings of their region's health care system. Stephen's case also illustrates the need for additional resources and facilities to treat PWAs. States that restrict PWAs from nursing and rest home facilities need to reevaluate their policies. As the disease continues to grow, additional health care facilities will be needed. For the HIV-infected person, group homes and limited-care living facilities are necessities. Additional financial resources are also needed to provide minimum levels of care for those who have contracted AIDS when the family actually cannot provide the help they need for medical care, housing, clothing, home care, food, and medicine.

Families With HIV-Infected Children Need Special Care

Seeing young infants and children with AIDS can be heart-breaking not only to the family but to the counselor or therapist as well. Parents and foster parents of children with AIDS need support groups that provide an understanding for what caring for a dying child means. Counselors can encourage mothers and foster mothers to take "time out" without feeling guilty. They can encourage fathers and foster fathers to participate more fully in the daily care of the child. Counselors can help parents prepare for feelings of loss and grief when the child dies. Many families with HIV-infected children rise to the occasion and find that not only do they love the child more, but they are stronger and more loving among themselves.

Marriages That Include a Person With AIDS Can Be Quite Strained

Many issues related to a husband or wife's serostatus can negatively affect a previously successful marriage. Knowledge of a partner's past (or current) drug use or extramarital sexual activities often results in feelings of anger and guilt. Often husbands and wives are reluctant to continue having sexual relations with each other based on their fear of contagion as in the following case.

Chuck was a drug user who was infected with HIV via a dirty needle. As his illness progressed, he lost the energy needed to work as an outdoor laborer. His wife began leaving him about once each month. When this occurred, he would move home with his parents for a day or two, work out a reconciliation with his wife, and move back into his home, only to bombard her with anger and hostility. In the marriage all sex was terminated and communication centered solely on the fact of Chuck's impending death. This resulted in his wife's feeling that Chuck did not love and care for her anymore. Chuck felt that he was a failure as a husband and was very ashamed of his disease.

Counselors can work with couples with infected members to facilitate more functional interactions. When wives are willing to support ailing husbands, counselors can help the couple see the change of traditional roles as a sign of love. Counselors can help couples find ways to avoid terminating all sexual sharing and instead practicing safer sex. Family counselors and therapists will need to be sensitive to the terrific sense of guilt that husbands and wives experience. Unless it is examined, this guilt will have an adverse effect on the couple's marriage.

All of the themes discussed above indicate that the person with AIDS, ARC, or other HIV infection needs the support of family and friends. The following 9 family support factors can be used by families with or without the guidance of a counselor to improve the quality of life for an infected person.

Family Support Factors

1. Family members should become familiar with social service agencies and the help that they provide for PWAs.
2. Family members and the PWA need to be open and honest in expressing their attitude toward this disease. Honesty seems to be the most important factor of continued open family communication.
3. If the family can afford therapy with a counselor, then the family and the PWA should be helped to deal with fear, guilt, and attitudes toward death.
4. A person with AIDS's partner/lover/spouse should always be included as a member of any family group whenever the family will tolerate this. The rights of spouses or lovers need to be guaranteed and their guilt and grief addressed.
5. Regardless of the past life style of the PWA, each PWA needs compassion and support. Families should view this disease as if it were any other life-threatening illness (i.e., cancer) and react with the same loving care that they would give to any dying member.
6. Regular contact with former friends and associates should be encouraged even when the PWA is very sick and dying. Often this is difficult for the family and friends of a PWA, but necessary for the maximal functioning of the dying person. Talking about the good times of life, planning for the funeral, making a will, and occasional bargaining with God for an immediate cure are

all a part of the struggle when persons find that they
must die. These tasks are often less painful when shared
with family members, lover(s), and friends.

7. Spiritual needs, which vary from person to person, need
to be respected. Compassionate clergy, desensitized to
AIDS, prove very helpful to the family, friends, and the
PWA.

8. Family members should help the PWA deal with the
realities of terminal illness. As long as the PWA feels
well enough, he or she should continue with former
activities and friends.

9. Family members and the PWA must learn to deal honestly with fear, anger, guilt, depression, and other related problems. In such dealings no one should take
personally things said or the panic that each person
occasionally feels. Families need to remember that an
honest, open, encouraging attitude will help everyone
involved, even when each is helpless. The person with
AIDS cannot change his or her disease. The family cannot change the disease. However, both the family and
the PWA can change the emotional context of their
attitudes toward AIDS if they will educate themselves
and deal honestly with it.

Implications for Family Therapists

It is important that family therapists as well as others in
the various helping professions realize that one of the effective
ways to help PWAs is through family-oriented therapy. No one
lives their life in a vacuum. The PWA may wish to conceal the
disease from family members in order to "protect" them from
its grim reality. However, in so doing, he or she still sends the
family messages that something is wrong. Although it is unlikely
that a family member can correctly anticipate the exact nature
of such atypical behavior, family members often have a general
sense that something is not right. For the most part, family
members can cope better with what they know, even if they do
not particularly like it, than with what they suspect.

In the family milieu there are those whose duty it is to
provide care for the dying. Families can rise to this occasion.
They can be most effective if they are helped by a therapist to

desensitize their fear of AIDS and become supportive. Families can be the primary care providers for PWAs and an effective home/family-based program of health care can prove vital to the needs of a person with AIDS.

If a family therapist helps the person with AIDS and his or her family members deal honestly with their emotions, the various stages of dying can be facilitated so there is a minimum of pain for those involved. This implies that no one can deny the realities of AIDS, ARC, or HIV seropositive status, no matter how attractive false hope or denial may seem to be. Family members and the PWA need to practice healthy emotional disclosure if they are to be functional. At the same time the anger and guilt that so often accompany this disease can be dealt with. Families need to be given permission to experience these feelings. In that way, they can grieve together and provide each other with social support as they deal with the death of a family member and, vicariously, with their own death.

As the disease progresses, there are often occasions when the patient will feel rather well, which creates false hope for the family. When the disease reoccurs, the patient and family may feel that they have been on a roller coaster. If families are to cope effectively with this prolonged illness, it is extremely important that they give each other brief intervals away from the situation where they can renew their coping abilities.

Conclusion

Family counselors and therapists see the person with AIDS, ARC, or HIV-positive serostatus and his or her family, be that parents, husband or wife, lovers or friends, as a system. In the face of AIDS, these systems need encouragement. As discussed in this chapter, the role of the family counselor or therapist is to join the family, act as a coach, encourage the family members, and demonstrate that he or she is unafraid of this disease. As a consequence, family counselors need to be desensitized to AIDS, drug use, homosexuality, prostitution, promiscuity, and a number of other related socially stigmatized behaviors. Once desensitized, the family therapist can provide the role model that helps family members and the PWA remain stable in the midst of this family crisis. The family therapist can help the family change so that they provide compassionate care and at the same time experience a closeness that reassures each member that he or she did all they could for their dying member. Such therapy is time-consuming, but it facilitates dying with dignity for the person with AIDS and caring with compassion for the family. Counseling that helps the infected person and his or her family members deal with their sense of loss, grief, and the realities of AIDS may be the most effective treatment available at this time.

With help, the family can be the resource that best helps the person with AIDS achieve a high quality of life after his or her diagnosis. Whether in a small nonmetropolitan region, where there are relatively few resources to help people with AIDS, or in large metropolitan centers, families are going to need on-going support, financial help, and encouragement. Family therapists, who prepare themselves to effectively educate and provide direct services to persons with AIDS, persons with ARC, or HIV infection, often with little financial reward, are doing pioneering work at the edge of this pandemic. In this work, every gain means hope for the people of the world for whom AIDS has become the feared disease of the 1980s and quite possibly the 1990s.

References

Brody, J.E. (1987, October 28). Personal hell. *New York Times*, offprint.

Carter, D.B. (1986). Aids and the sex therapist: "Just the facts please Ma'am." *Journal of Sex Research, 22,* 403–408.

Curtis, J.H., & Richardson, M.M. (1986). *The epidemiology of AIDS in Georgia: An analysis of statistical projections for Georgia, metropolitan Atlanta, and each Georgia county 1985–2000.* Unpublished research report.

Forum. (1987, September-October). The impact of AIDS on death education, counseling, and care. Santa Cruz, CA: *Newsletter of the Association for Death Education and Counseling.*

Mohr, R. (1988). Deciding what's do-able. *The Family Therapy Networker, 22,* 34–36.

Morin, S.F., & Batchelor, W.F. (1984). Responding to the psychological crisis of AIDS. *Public Health Reports, 99,* 4–9.

Nichols, M.P. (1984). *Family therapy: Concepts and methods.* New York: Gardner Press.

Patten, J. (1988, January/February). AIDS and the gay couple. *The Family Therapy Networker, 12,* 37–39.

Richardson, M.M., & Curtis, J.H. (1986). *Predicted AIDS-related deaths in Georgia: 1985–2000*. Unpublished research report.

Simon, R. (1988, January/February). AIDS and family therapy. *The Family Therapy Networker, 12*, 33.

Walker, G. (1988, January/February). An AIDS journal. *The Family Therapy Networker 12*, 20–32.

Chapter 10

MODERN HOSPICE CARE

Sr. Patrice Murphy and Carole Donovan

When a person becomes seriously ill, there comes a time when no further treatment can be offered to reverse the ravages of the disease. What is needed are measures to promote comfort, to alleviate such symptoms as nausea and diarrhea, and to prepare for a peaceful death. In short, what is needed is hospice care—a health care approach that embraces and supports the patient without searching for unobtainable cures. Hospice care traditionally was offered to persons who suffered from cancer or other illnesses in which a 6-month prognosis could be determined. With the emergence of the AIDS epidemic it became clear that those afflicted with AIDS could benefit greatly from receiving hospice care.

In 1967, St. Christopher's Hospice in Sydenham, England, opened its doors to terminally ill persons who had cancer and began a revolution in health care. Dame Cecily Saunders, its founder, believed that care at St. Christopher's ". . . should stem from respect for the patient and very close attention to his distress . . . to plan and carry out research in the relief of distress such as has not been done anywhere else" (Saunders, 1965, p. 1615). St. Christopher's demonstrated that patients could be helped to live to the fullest—even when death was only hours away.

It was through the work at St. Christopher's that pain relief without severe drowsiness became a reality. Studies carried out there demonstrated that an analgesic titrated to the degree of a person's pain could eliminate that pain most of the time yet enable the person to participate in the life around him or her.

Although St. Christopher's opened its doors 21 years ago, hospice care is not a new concept. The term hospice originally described a stopping place for pilgrims in medieval times. In this country it has come to represent a type of care rather than a place of care. That is, it is care that is concerned with making patients comfortable so that they can continue to live as fully as possible in the remaining time of their life. Pain is controlled, nausea subdued, appetite encouraged, weakness supported. Hospice care is generally provided to terminally ill persons whose prognosis is estimated at 6 months or less. The care can be provided in a free-standing facility, in a hospital, or in the patient's home. The first hospice program in this country was The Connecticut Hospice, Inc. in Brandford, which began providing care in 1974. Currently there are over 1,600 hospice programs throughout the United States. Of these, 625 are Medicare certified. States vary in their requirements concerning licensure.

With the increasing numbers of persons infected with the human immunodeficiency virus (HIV) and ill with AIDS, it became clear that hospice care was an appropriate part of their health care. In a report to Health and Welfare Canada, the Expert Working Group on Integrated Palliative Care for Persons with AIDS stated that ". . . as the present outcome is always fatal and much shorter than cancer care in general, preparation and integration for death should begin at diagnosis" (1987, p.16). Thus, while active aggressive care can be directed toward controlling symptoms and disease, those issues concerning the eventual death of the patient are, therefore, incorporated into the early care of the person with AIDS. Such issues include informing others of the patient's terminal illness, expressing the patient's grief concerning his or her losses and impending death, completing a will, and designating someone to have power of attorney and durable power of attorney.

The Supportive Care Program at St. Vincent's Hospital and Medical Center in New York City began working with AIDS patients in late 1983. The staff decided that patients who had AIDS could be accepted at any point in their illness when the Supportive Care team could be helpful. The usual hospice guideline of a 6-month prognosis was not imposed because it was not clear how this timeframe could be determined in these patients. The illness and its course were entirely unpredictable. Often by taking patients into the program at what turns out to be an early state of their illness has been valuable. The staff have come to know the patient and his or her coping styles when illness has not been overwhelming.

Modern comprehensive hospice care is composed of basic tenets. These tenets include: patient and family are the unit of care; care is managed by an interdisciplinary team; trained volunteers supplement and complement the efforts of professional staff; focus of care is on symptom management; hospice care is available on a 24-hour, 7-day-week basis; and bereavement care is available to loved ones after the patient's death.

Patient and Family—The Unit of Care

For persons with AIDS (PWAs) the term family is frequently broadly defined. Some have strong ties with their family of origin as well as significant relationships with carefully chosen others. Others may have moved away from their parents' house at an early age because they were aware of being "different" and of needing to seek the closeness and companionship of others like themselves; this is frequently true of the gay PWA. Although these individuals may maintain cordial realtions with parents and siblings, they often share little about their personal lives and life styles or may share this information with only one family member.

Still others have been rejected by parents or siblings because of their homosexuality or use of drugs. Attempts at reconciliation by sons or daughters may have been fruitless. Disappointment, sadness, and anger mount on each side.

A small percentage of PWAs are individuals who initially denied their gay sexual orientation and pursued a heterosexual life style—often marrying and fathering children—only to find at some point that they could no longer live a lie and subsequently were impelled to seek a divorce. Another small percentage of PWAs, whose numbers are growing rapidly, are those who have become infected because of an IV drug history, and who, in turn, are infecting wives or girl friends and their infants. Confusion, shock, fear, and rage are emotions frequently experienced by family members of such persons if or when the infected individuals reveal their situation. A small percentage of PWAs are bisexual and their extramarital sexual activities have led to their infection. Finally, there are those PWAs who have contracted the disease because they received transfusions infected with the HIV.

When hospice workers speak of family and people with AIDS, they are talking about those with family created by blood relation, those created by the individual's choice, and those created solely of the professionals or paraprofessionals caring for the patient. Hospice workers supporting PWAs and their families are not only dealing with the patient's terminal illness, but with a myriad of charged issues and emotions of family members including homophobia, fear of contagion, shock, guilt, shame, anger, sorrow, secrecy, and ambivalence. Availability of hospice staff to family members for discussing issues, sharing emotions, and confronting fears and ambivalence is of major importance in the care of both patient and family. Often hospice staffs, by their warm and caring actions and attitudes toward the patient, serve as role models to those loved ones who are uncertain or fearful in their approach to the patient.

It is not uncommon for many parents to learn that their son is gay at the same time they learn that he has AIDS. Jack, for example, did not want to tell his burly truck-driving dad that he had AIDS and that his illness was related to his gay life style. His mother urged him to include his dad in the sharing of this information as did his hospice nurse. When Jack did, his father responded, "You're my son. I love you no matter what." Tom, on the other hand, called his dad to inform him about his diagnosis and to ask for some financial help. On hearing about Tom's diagnosis, his dad replied, "The wages of sin are death." That was the last Tom heard from his father.

Peter called St. Vincent's to ask for help in working with his sister. Peter, who was 38 years old, had been diagnosed a year before with Kaposi's sarcoma (KS). Like Rock Hudson, he had been treated in Paris, but without success. His KS lesions most severely affected his face. His eyes were nearly closed because of the extensive swelling of his lids. His nose was large, almost bulblike and black. In fact, it looked as though someone had replaced the tip with a large black olive.

Peter's lover had left him the fall Peter was diagnosed as having AIDS. That Christmas, Peter was to spend the holiday with his sister, Judy. He called to tell her his diagnosis. Judy called him back and told him that he could not visit for the holiday. In fact, he could not visit in her home at all. Her husband had recently recovered from a serious illness and did not feel secure about having Peter there.

Peter was anguished and angry. He wanted the hospice team's help because he feared that Judy would be guilt-ridden following his death. They had always had a close relationship.

Both parents had died and they were all that remained of their family. The nurse who visited Peter listened to his concerns and to his anger about Judy. She spoke with Judy and heard her anguish at not being able to be with Peter. Judy's husband would allow Judy to visit Peter, but only if they met in a public place, not Peter's apartment, and Judy was not to touch him. Judy felt a deep conflict between her love for her husband and love for her brother. To help work out some of the issues of forgiveness and conflict, the nurse arranged for a young priest who volunteered with the program to meet with Peter.

In time Peter was able to say that he forgave Judy. Judy was able to put aside her conflicts and meet Peter and hug him. Although Peter had a number of physical problems that required attention, it was really the issue of his relationship to Judy that troubled him most. When that work was complete, Peter arranged to have one last weekend in the Catskills with his friends. He wanted to see a starry sky, to play Trivial Pursuit, and savor a world he was ready to leave. When the weekend was over, his friends had to piggyback an exhausted, weakened Peter up the stairs to his apartment. Within 2 days, Peter died quietly in his sleep.

Conflicts between the PWA and his or her family may ultimatley never be resolved. Those PWAs and their families affiliated with a hospice program whose staff is prepared, skilled, and sensitive to the possible wide range of family reactions, reap the benefits of the efforts of these professionals and volunteers. Not infrequently, patients and families face death reconciled and peaceful.

Hospice Care is Managed by an Interdisciplinary Team

Physicians, nurses, social workers, pastoral care persons, and trained volunteers make up the core hospice team. Many of these individuals have devoted themselves to hospice work out of a sense of frustration and dissatisfaction with the limitations of institutional care of the terminally ill and a cogent desire to use their skills and talents to improve this situation for others. By working together with a sense of interdependence, they found they were better able to share and coordinate their philosophies and goals of care and thus more fully meet the manifold needs of the terminally ill patient and family. When the individual team members respect and appreciate one another's expertise and special gifts of mind and spirit, and when conflicts are recognized and resolved quickly, the team is not only a source of strength and support for patients and families but also for one another. This is no small advantage.

The roles of hospice physician, nurse, social worker, and chaplain are familiar to most people, but the role of the volunteer in the service and support of the terminally ill is less well recognized. Volunteers have been the backbone of hospice care since its inception in the United States and are unique among those rendering services to patients and families. What do hospice volunteers do? The possibilities are endless. Volunteers can visit a patient, read to him or her, take the patient for a walk, for coffee, to a movie or a play, bring the wheelchair-bound patient for a ride outdoors, cook a meal, listen empathetically, explore issues with the patient or family, comfort family members, and provide respite for caregivers. The occasions for volunteers to be a caring presence to the patients and families are as many and varied as the individuals involved.

Volunteers do what they do because of a desire to serve in a way that is not concerned with the usual problems of earning a living. They have special and unusual motivation; a price tag cannot be attached to their special gifts of self and service. Volunteers humanize services by extending and enriching the care rendered by staff whose duties often do not allow them time to provide the "extras" that often they wish they could offer. There will never be enough people to meet the deep human needs of the sick and dying and their loved ones.

The increase of individuals interested in assisting PWAs has occurred steadily since the beginning of the AIDS crisis. Many large communities have developed a variety of volunteer groups, and hospice is a setting chosen by many volunteers for their services to PWAs. However, a volunteer program costs money. Recruiting, screening, training, supervising, and supporting volunteers is expensive when done well, but the finished product justifies the price. Volunteers to PWAs and their loved ones have proved to be a priceless ingredient of the total blend that constitutes hospice care.

In a hospice team there are times when roles may blur. A social worker may notice a change in a patient's way of relating or a physical manifestation previously unnoted that may herald the beginning of a new symptom. Hospice nurses may find themselves counseling patients and loved ones and establishing in-depth realtionshps. Hospice chaplains often find themselves advocating for patients' rights. Blurring of roles is all to the good, and where team members are united in their philosophies and goals, such role blurring can result in maximizing support and comfort for patients and loved ones.

Pastoral care can often be an area of role blurring because all team members are involved in responding to the spiritual side of their patients. In approaching patients and loved ones with a deep respect for the intrinsic value of each human being and a nonjudgmental acceptance of the person as unique, caregivers are responding to the most basic spiritual need of all human beings. Often respect and acceptance of this quality serve as a foundation for further work by patient and pastoral counselors in facing the issues and needs that emerge when patients are confronting death.

Persons with AIDS do not always raise existential questions with the hospice chaplain or pastoral counselor. Nurses, social workers, and even volunteers may be confronted with questions or statements such as: "Why is this happening to me? I never hurt anyone." "Is God angry with me?" "Some people say I brought this all on myself." "What is dying like?" "Will I be brave enough?" "I'm not afraid of death, but I'm afraid of dying." Sometimes there aren't responses to these statements or answers to the questions. At other times, exploring with the patient who his or her God is and what his or her life journey has been like thus far may facilitate a discussion whereby the patient will arrive at his or her own answers. It is always helpful for the caregiver to reassure the patient that hospice staff members will do everything possible to relieve pain or other bothersome symptoms whenever they occur.

Are we, as professional caregivers, as members of a team, ready for such questions? We are if, in working with terminally ill persons and their loved ones, we have learned to face our own mortality, if we have examined the fears and hope in our own hearts and spirits, if we are in touch with the depths of our own beliefs, and if we believe that each person's spirituality, including that of the caregiver, is unique yet always involved with relationships—relationship to self, relationship to others, and ultimately relationship to God or whoever God is for the individual.

Hospice Availability: 24 Hours—7 Days per Week

This tenet of hospice care is a difficult and often costly one. The ideal being sought by this requirement is continuity of professional care and caring, that is, the availability of hospice-prepared individuals on a continuing basis, uninterrupted by the closing of offices and weekend or holiday breaks. Each program, true to its commitment to comprehensive hospice care, must seek out its own method of best responding to this tenet of care. Examples of meeting this prescription have been the utilization of carefully trained and highly motivated professional volunteers who take turns being "on call" during each month, or the hiring of per diem staff for the hospice whose sole responsibility is being "on call" after hours and on weekends and holidays, particularly for those hospice patients who are in their own homes.

Despite the difficulties involved in meeting this particular criterion, instances where patients and loved ones have used this service prove its importance to both the physical and emotional well-being of the patient and loved ones. Patients with AIDS who often have high anxiety levels may find themselves panicked by a change or increase in a symptom such as a rise in temperature. Vulnerable and emotionally drained loved ones may find they need the reassurance and support of a caring hospice professional. Often telephone contact will serve as the means of soothing or providing directions or explanation. Listening may be the most effective therapy a patient or loved one can receive. Some calls may require a visit from the "on-call" person in order to assess the situation, and some situations may require the professional "on-call" person to be the liaison between the patient and physician or pharmacy or volunteer, depending on the circumstances and the outcome of the assessment. It is significant how often this service has meant the difference between maintaining a patient at home rather than rushing him or her to an emergency room where impersonal and sometimes highly technical modalities of treatment not desired by the patient or loved ones may be utilized. Whatever the need—be it only a patient's need to check that there is truly someone "on call"— strength and caring is communicated to the caller.

Sometimes a call may come to the "on-call" person from a loved one saying that he or she thinks that the patient is dying or has died. Shock, sorrow, and confusion may be evident in the caller's voice, and the response of the alert, caring "on-call" hospice person can make a tremendous difference in how a patient or loved ones face and respond to this event and how the memory of that powerful experience will affect them in the future.

Management of Symptoms

The hospice movement vigorously stands against the aseptic walling off of the terminally ill patient from him- or herself and from other human beings. Rather, it offers a carefully designed program of "loving care" where all caregivers are sensitively attuned to recognizing and responding to the needs and the rights of the terminally ill (Anderson & MacElveen-Hoehn, 1988). Needs may include affirmation and validation of decisions, privacy, independence, and the desire to continue living life as normally as possible. Rights often include being included in all plans for one's own care and treatment, receiving full information regarding options available in treatment, or stopping treatment as well as continuing it.

Expertise in managing pain is perhaps the best recognized contribution of the hospice concept and philosophy to terminal care. Because oral preparations and rectal suppositories of many effective pain medications are available in local pharmacies, it is frequently possible to work out pain control in the patient's home. Some pain medications are available in time-release capsules whereby relief is spread over long time periods. Hospice team members are knowledgeable about dosage and side effects and readily recognize untoward symptoms that may indicate an unwelcome side effect of a medication. It is often this specialized knowledge and expertise that has gained hospice care its recognition and acceptance with patients, families, and physicians.

Persons with AIDS tend to have many symptoms during the course of their disease process, and their management can be complex. Discussion of symptoms begins with their unpredictability. Thereafter, consideration of symptomatology entails familiarity with each body system. For the purpose of this chapter, discussion of symptoms is limited to unpredictability, anxiety, depression, and suicide.

Unpredictability

To take on the care of PWAs is to take on uncertainty. Most hospice staffs have grown familiar with the terminal illnesses from which patients in their programs die. They have accumulated data on the course of diseases and the probable impact that appropriate treatments or their lack will have on the trajectory of the illness. Hospice staffs are able to anticipate difficulties and often prevent them because collective experience has sharpened their sensitivity and intuition. With AIDS the scenario is very different. There is no long history of experience in managing the disease, and therefore, there is a decreased comfort level for the professional caregivers. Some symptoms and the processes causing them are rare and occur without warning, such as spontaneous pneumothorax (collapsed lung) and cardiac tamponade (compression of the heart that can lead to standstill), and require acute and intensive management in hospital. Other symptoms are frequent and apparently simple to treat, but these treatments present varying levels of difficulty and success. Among these are a fungal infection (thrush) in the mouth or esophagus, chronic diarrhea, fever, anorexia, and dehydration. Tumors such as those of the walls of blood vessels (known as Kaposi's sarcoma) can cause problems in many different parts of the body—skin, oral mucosa, palate, gastrointestinal tract, lungs, liver, and spleen. Sometimes these occur concurrently. Whenever and wherever these occur, they challenge the knowledge, understanding, and ingenuity of the most skilled caregivers. Although Kaposi's sarcoma may be the more common malignancy seen in PWAs, non-Hodgkins lymphoma, an aggressive malignant tumor that can be found anywhere from rectum to abdominal cavity, from chest wall to nasal septum to brain, is all too frequently diagnosed in persons with AIDS. Both chemotherapy and radiation therapy have been used in treatment. Response has varied; no treatment has eliminated the tumors, which alone or in combination with opportunistic infections, lead to the death of these patients.

Among the infections that occur in these patients are those caused by protozoa. Pneumocystis carinii pneumonia (PCP) can be an insidious or rapidly progressing lung infection. Toxoplasmosis can cause an infection in the brain or lead to visual loss. Crytosporidiosis is commonly known as traveler's diarrhea, but may be more persistent in the PWA. Cytomegalovirus is a herpes virus that can affect the eyes, liver, lungs, and brain. These diseases can often be treated but never cured. Many treatments have their own set of complications that can also be debilitating and even life-threatening, such as low white blood cell count (neutropenia), a low platelet count (thrombocytopenia), severe skin reactions, high or low glucose levels, and renal damage.

Anxiety

The threat of exposure to the HIV virus and the fear it inspires have forced people to develop a variety of coping mechanisms ranging from denial to substantial adaptation. When coping mechanisms are inadequate, fear may increase to the point where it can become irrational and prompt maladaptive behaviors that are debilitating and destructive.

Most of the research to date on anxiety and depression in PWAs has been with the gay or bisexual population. Intravenous drug abusers, who have their own special problems, do not usually find their way to private or clinic therapy or into reseach studies. Many PWAs experience guilt and shame and expect punishment; they may feel anger and resentment toward other gay individuals suspected of infecting them. There may also be a simultaneous concern and regret for other PWAs for whose infection they may feel responsible. Shame and guilt contribute to serious loss of self-esteem that in turn may lead to social withdrawal, an increase in depression, and even suicide.

In an article entitled "Psychotherapy and the AIDS-Anxious Patient," C. Richard Filson and Charles R. Tartaglia (1988) concluded:

> "... Despite the shifts in the issues patients face after diagnosis, problems maintaining self-esteem, retaining a clear sense of identity, finding meaning in day to day activities, holding on to important relationships, preserving a sense of control often require a therapist's assistance .... active engagement of the patient, understanding the meaning of symptoms (such as fear of death or disability) and determining psychological characteristics and coping styles are techniques which can help therapists in their efforts to provide care. (p. 2)

Depression and Suicide

In a recently published study of suicide in persons with AIDS in New York City, Marzuk, Tierney, and Tardiff (1988) provided the first epidemiologic documentation for a distinct relationship between AIDS and the act that, above all others, signals desperation and hopelessness—suicide. The study indicates that in 1985 the rate of suicide among New York City residents with AIDS (614 deaths per 100,000 persons per year) was 66 times higher than that of the general population of New York City. Men 20–59 years of age with an AIDS diagnosis were 36 times as likely to commit suicide as were men in the general population of New York City. The authors note that it is likely that these figures underestimate the true AIDS-related suicide rate.

These facts confirm the suspicion of many professional caregivers of persons with AIDS and reinforce the need for physicians, nurses, social workers, and pastoral counselors to explore openly the issues of suicide where the risk of suicide is suspected. The patient with overwhelming feelings of panic, guilt, shame, depression, and hopelessness, and the one with the neurological complications of delirium or dementia are acknowledged to be at high risk for suicide.

Preventive measures to reduce the risk of suicide are similar to those used with patients suffering from other serious illnesses. Opportunities for open discussion of feeling surrounding diagnosis; fears of disability, deterioration, and ultimately death; guilt over fractured but important relationships or over the embarrassment caused loved ones; and frustrated desires to retain some control over their lives are crucial issues for "at-risk" patients to explore with trained hospice team members.

Neuropsychiatric consultations must be sought where there is evidence of complications such as marked depression, dementia, or delirium. Such complications should be assessed and treated in order, if at all possible, to maximize the quality of the patient's life. Marzuk et al. (1988) stated, "Caring for patients whose illnesses bring them to the painful extremes of human experience has always been one of the most challenging aspects of the physician's role." This statement can be equally true for hospice nurses, social workers, pastoral caregivers, and volunteers.

When one reflects on the array of possible symptoms that the person with AIDS may manifest, there seem to be three primary courses that the disease may take and of which each hospice team member needs to be aware. Severe sudden opportunistic infections such as pneumocystis carinii pneumonia and death; gradual decline with periods of relative stability between acute episodes; and lastly, a course characterized by a combination of the other two such as an acute sudden first illness, gradual decline, and then an unexpected death during a period of what was thought to be stability.

Sudden unexpected deaths are not the norm in hospice care. Usually there are clear signals that a patient's condition is deteriorating; loved ones and staff have an opportunity to say final goodbyes. With AIDS, unexpected and sudden deaths occur with some regularity and are upsetting to everyone involved. Such rapid, unanticipated, irreversible decline adds to the level of fear, powerlessness, and uncertainty for all.

Timmy is an example of a patient in the last category. The hospice team at St. Vincent's met him in the hospital during his initial opportunistic infection of PCP. Timmy was in his 30s, had come to the mainland United States from Hawaii where his parents and sibling lived. He was an unusual man with a winning smile. Even in the throes of a 105-degree fever and severe shaking chills he never complained. Timmy had a special friend with whom he lived and he worried about him. Always, his concern was more for his friend than himself; when with his hospice caregivers, he would always try to divert their attention away from himself toward his friend. Although most of the hospice teams' experience with Timmy was in his home, he required hospital admission on two occasions for unexplained fevers. During the last admission, when he was not in bed with fever and chills, Timmy was ambulatory, visiting some patients confined to their rooms and chatting with others in the lounge. He was much loved by staff and fellow patients. During the night following a relatively comfortable day, the nurses on their rounds found Timmy pulseless and not breathing. Emergency resuscitation efforts failed to bring him back to life. A great sadness descended upon staff and patients on Timmy's unit and on the hospice staff who had cared for him at home.

Symptom management is no less a challenge to the social worker or pastoral care provider on the hospice staff than it is for the hospice physician or nurse. Patient and family comfort levels are only satisfactorily addressed when each team member's goal is excellence in assessment, observation, sensitivity, communication, and intervention.

Bereavement Care

Bereavement services complete the continuum of care provided by hospice caregivers to the patient's loved ones. Services are offered after careful assessment of the needs of the primary griever(s) and with great respect for the individuality and desires of those grieving. These services can be as simple as a periodic phone call to ask "How are you? We're thinking about you." They can be more structured, with regularly planned phone calls by a staff member or a volunteer, or they may take the form of participation in a bereavement support self-help group. However, it is most important to realize that bereavement services ideally begin prior to death with both the patient (if this is possible and appropriate) and with loved ones. Grief work that begins before the patient's death is called anticipatory grieving.

The Patient

We all, as caregivers, recognize that grief and mourning are a normal and appropriate response to loss, but not everyone acknowledges that the terminally ill person also grieves. For patients with AIDS, grief may begin with the diagnosis and further intensify as the disease progresses. The accumulation of losses for these patients with AIDS can be great depending on the length and degree of illness. Physical appearance, youth, and beauty are highly valued in our culture, especially in the gay subculture. PWAs grieve the loss of their appearance. Handsome young people with special gifts of charm and sensitivity gradually, or sometimes quickly, lose the appearance of which they were so proud. Significant weight loss, muscle wasting, thinning of hair, dramatic purplish lesions, fatigue, and listlessness lead to drastic changes in appearance, and often the once-handsome young person may be barely recognizable or not recognizable at all. Society is learning that having an appearance that resembles a walking skeleton or a concentration camp prisoner can be a telltale sign of AIDS; this may make public activites awkward and uncomfortable for PWAs. It may mean loss of livelihood. The fatigue associated with AIDS can be overwhelming and often precipitates lateness for work, absences, and inability to produce as effectively as previously.

Eventually, the patient must confront his or her inability to continue to hold down a job. Loss of job heralds loss of income, perhaps also the ending of insurance coverage. The PWA with gradually diminishing resources becomes dependent on the goodness and generosity of relatives, friends, or the entitlements available at city and state levels.

All too frequently PWAs face the loss of relatives and friends. Family members—shocked, ashamed, and righteous—may completely reject or withdraw coolly so that their emotional involvement in the plight of the PWA is negligible. Friends, often young, frightened, vulnerable, and confused, may withdraw gradually but noticeably. The patient's grief deepens. These losses have profound implications for the sick person because the caring presence and attentiveness of loved ones, even in the face of terrible debility and impending death, is a source of hope and comfort to the dying patient.

Just as counselors have roles in society, in professions, in family, so too, did those now diagnosed with AIDS. When an actor can no longer act, or an artist can no longer paint, or a physician can no longer heal, his or her concept of self diminishes. Hopelessness may follow.

Loss of life—one's own— can be incomprehensible to the young PWA. Usually young people in their 20s and 30s have had little life experience with significant personal loss. Perhaps a grandparent with whom he or she felt close ties has died, but even that contributes little to preparing a young person for his or her own death. At an age when most young people feel immortal, and society—a death and grief denying society— perpetuates that myth, PWAs have usually never even imagined dealing with their own death.

Looking at death at any age clearly is not easy. Some PWAs seem to operate on two levels when talking about their death. On one level, they believe and hope they will survive long enough to see a cure found. They seek out alternative therapies such as healing groups, acupuncture, and diet as a way to stave off death. They look to returning to work as a way to confirm that life is going to go on as before. On another level, they prepare their wills and assign power of attorney. Somewhere in the progression of their illness, they begin to accept that physical losses will not reverse and that death ultimately will be the outcome of their disease.

What moves a patient toward understanding that he or she will die from the disease is unclear. Surely being emotionally supported by a caregiver who listens, who suggests measures to alleviate symptoms, who cares, provides the safe environment in which even the most terrifying events can be considered.

Confronting death is often as difficult for the parents, siblings, lovers, and close friends of the PWA as it is for him or her. Not only is it difficult to confront death, it is also difficult to express one's grief in a society that has little sympathy for those who have contracted AIDS. The survivors—the family, friends, and lovers—often become "hidden grievers."

Loved Ones

Experiences with these grieving individuals have demonstrated the terrible isolation and secrecy with which loved ones often surround themselves, closing themselves off to the supports ordinarily available for those who grieve. Often they respond in this way because they are frightened. Parents frequently tell no one the truth about their child's death. They fear that the truth could mean loss of their support systems because of the stigma of AIDS, fear of contagion, and moralistic reasons. They live a lie and grieve quietly and alone.

Lovers and close friends are "hidden grievers" because they also are afraid—afraid of the fallout for themselves—if people knew the depths of their grief and its reasons. They are afraid of losing their jobs or apartments or business associates, afraid of overburdening their friends and causing them to withdraw, and afraid for their own health or lack of health. They are in the midst of a process they can barely define let alone acknowledge.

Grief is a normal, natural, and lengthy process; it has a beginning, middle, and end. Young people, new to grief experiences and enmeshed in an "instant" society, are ill prepared for the devastating pain and loneliness of loss and for the tasks of mourning that need to be accomplished before healthy resolution can occur.

The experienced practitioners in a hospice program, where grief in all its manifestations is recognized and acknowledged, can play a significant role in the lives of the various "hidden grievers." Hospice staff working through the grief process with the bereaved either on a one-to-one basis or in a group setting, find that those grieving often discover that working through grief, despite its terrible pain, can become a significant factor in individual growth and development. Many reach new depths of humanity and spirituality when they are assisted in their grief work to accomplish the tasks of mourning. Lastly, we look at the grief of those who have been the hospice caregivers in the hospital, the clinic, or at home.

The Caregiver

The term "hidden grievers" encompasses another group of individuals of whose grief others have little awareness. They are the hospice nurses, physicians, social workers, counselors, and volunteers who have spent much time with PWAs. Society doesn't think of professional caregivers as individuals who often experience a deep sense of loss when a patient with AIDS for whom they have cared and grown to appreciate, and even love, dies. Professionals are considered the "strong" ones, people prepared by some special curriculum to face dying and death, even if it occurs several times in a 24-hour period, with equilibrium, even detachment. The reality is that caregivers are, first and foremost, human beings who are often deeply concerned and committed to working with patients with AIDS. Frequently these caregivers have chosen to care for people with AIDS. For these caregivers, hospice care means not intensive technological care but intensive people care. With PWAs, this intensive people care is further augmented by the bonds that are created between a caregiver and patient who is confronting his or her death. Helping people with AIDS face the losses inherent in the progression of their illness means sharing intimate moments with special people. Lannie (1984) wrote that "anguish is always present when we are forced to say goodbye" (p. 33). It is present for the PWA and it is present for the caregiver.

Working with the dying and the bereaved can touch caregivers personally in several ways. Such work can reawaken pain over personal losses, increase apprehension regarding potential losses in the caregiver's own life, and perhaps bring to awareness troubling feelings about the caregiver's own mortality. Feeling helpless in the presence of a disease that always ends in death can be debilitating and depressing.

This very pain of grief, however, can contain for the caregiver the potential for growth. Often it is in the midst of sorrow that we are forced to take time to assess the meaning of our own lives, evaluate our priorities of living, and, perhaps, experience the real substance of life. Sometimes it is our grief that helps us to realize the difference between existing and living.

Implications for Caregivers

AIDS patients, unlike any other patients we have encountered, are generally aware that their illness has no cure at present and will ultimately end in death. One must be aware that patients slip in and out of denial about their illness, about whether they will "beat the odds." Gentleness is needed when the patient seeks comfort for a brief while in self-deception. One must not push toward reality. A physician, for example, who thought it best to lay forth to the patient the new results of some diagnostic work told him that what he had was an overwhelming cryptococcal infection and that his life expectancy was now 4 weeks. The nurse came upon the patient shortly after this disclosure and found a young man struggling to hold himself together. While she was there, an intern who came in to draw his blood said, upon leaving the room, that he would be back in 10 minutes to answer some questions the patient had. In fury the patient screamed, "Do you know how long 10 minutes is for someone who has only 4 weeks?"

In working with these patients, one must be alert to the issues that surround dying and death—the need to say good-byes, to tidy up one's affairs, to reflect on one's life, and to come to terms with how that life has been. The caregiver must be comfortable with confronting these issues with the patient. The patient is not looking for answers for the most part but, rather, is looking to be heard, to have someone tolerate the expressions of fear, anxiety, and pain concerning what he or she is about to lose. It is the honest responses, the willingness to explore the ending of a life as one does the beginning or middle that makes it possible for the patient to relinquish his or her anxieties and move toward a peaceful closure in life. Moving a person toward that peace is the most caring, the most loving approach that one human being can offer another.

Conclusion

Not every person with AIDS will elect hospice services nor is hospice care advocated for all people with AIDS. Our hope is that the reader will be able to appreciate that hospice care is a viable option for PWAs and that many such persons and their loved ones have benefited and will continue to benefit from its philosophy and how it is played out in relation to the multitude of problems and issues inherent in this dreaded illness. In Rossman (1979), Edmund Pellegrino, M.D., Director of the Kennedy Institute of Ethics, summarizes the value of the hospice concept and philosophy to all terminally ill persons in the following words:

> . . . The challenges for medical, nursing and health profession educators are direct, specific and inescapable as they are for administrators, boards of trustees and public policy makers. The ideal of patient-oriented, patient-centered, and patient-directed medical care is, perhaps, the most difficult unmet challenge before us today . . . . the hospice movement alerts all of us to a signal deficiency which no amount of elaborate technology, systems organization, or managerial efficiency can obliterate. Only persons can care, and without caring even the hospice idea becomes just another formula. (p. 8)

References

Anderson, H., & MacElveen-Hoehn, T. (1988). Gay clients with AIDS: New challenges for hospice programs. *The Hospice Journal, 4*, 37–54.

Expert Working Group on Integrative Palliative Care for Persons with AIDS. (1988, Dec.). *AIDS care—Basic reference information for the preparation of community AIDS plan* (condensation of *Caring Together* report to Health and Welfare Canada), p. 16.

Filson, C.R., & Tartaglia, C.R. (1988). Psychotherapy and the AIDS-anxious patient. *Focus—A Guide to AIDS Research, 3*, 2.

Lannie, V.J. (1984, Fall). The positive aspects of anguish. *American Journal of Hospice Care*, pp. 33–35.

Marzuk, P.M., Tierney, H., & Tardiff, K. (1988). Increased risk of suicide in persons with AIDS. *The Journal of the American Medical Association, 259*, 1333–1337.

Rossman, P. (1979). *Hospice*. Piscataway, NJ: New Century Publishers.

Saunders, C. (1965). Watch with me. *Nursing Times, 61*, 1615.

Chapter 11

SUSTAINING THE SPIRIT

Rev. Albert J. Ogle

Jim Cotter, a theologian from England, described the ancient and still practiced custom of building "cairns" with stone on lonely mountain paths to mark some special, significant places (1987). People would merely add a stone to the existing pile as they journeyed on the way to the next marker in search of the journey's end. There is comfort and hope in the knowledge that other human beings, bewildered, tired, challenged, and caring have gone this way before; the "cairn" represents something of a collective consciousness and solidarity with fellow travelers. AIDS presents counselors with an opportunity to contribute to the existing markers on the paths from birth to death. When the AIDS crisis is over, which stories or memorials will remain? What can be learned from those who have died? This chapter shares experiences, ideas, and strategies for counselors and their clients when looking at spiritual issues that emerge as part of the AIDS crisis.

AIDS: A Crisis for the Counselor

One of the most powerful feelings associated with AIDS is isolation. Legislation, special health care programs, and attitudes in society either isolate the person with AIDS or integrate him or her. This is also done to people in leadership positions in health and psychosocial care of AIDS patients, for example, counselors. Counselors need to ask, "Am I feeling isolated in my AIDS work or integrated?" Counselors will only be really effective as they integrate themselves and their clients into a "family-like" model that is truly our natural *support system*. Rabbi Edwin Friedman's book *Generation to Generation* (1987), although basically a handbook for pastors of congregations, gives a useful approach in how to work with crisis situations in families and congregations utilizing a family systems model. This model can also help counselors and therapists be effective in their work and avoid burnout.

Friedman's (1987) basic thesis is that as a community "healer," a counselor cannot isolate a family, congregational, or client's crisis from his or her own interior work. Counselors must contemplate why they are working with AIDS patients. What issues in their own life and value system surface for them as a result of AIDS? It may be that the counselor is gay, that the counselor identifies with younger people suffering and dying, that the counselor has lost a close friend or family member, or that the counselor feels a moral imperative to "do" something. Whatever has "dragged" counselors into the AIDS experience needs to be owned and clearly defined if counselors are to be effective. Friedman uses the term "self-differentiation" to describe the need to own one's own issues and differentiate from the external crisis. If the congregational leader or counselor isn't aware of his or her own direction, goals, or motives, there is little hope that the counselor will be of much use in helping a person with AIDS, a family, or a community understand or love themselves more fully.

The personal challenge to all people engaged in AIDS-related work is how to balance professional and personal "self-differentiation" with owning one's issues that are stimulated by people with HIV and AIDS. There is much work for counselors to do with people who come to them for help and meaning in their lives, and their process often stimulates the counselors' own. Counselors can be effective only in as much as they recognize and develop their own growth. The mental health profession is having to face deep dark questions that are, in essence, profoundly spiritual. For example, the chapter's author recently conducted an inservice training on AIDS for special education teachers in Los Angeles. It was difficult work, highly demanding, low paying, and not significantly recognized by the community at large. It was engaging for the author to relate his experience of working with persons with AIDS with working with their population. They had chosen to involve themselves deeply with members of society who have been ostracized and largely ignored, and yet they loved their work and the people they served. "Vocation" is a word that is intimately connected to the word "profession." To profess is to *believe* that you want to and are skilled enough to do a particular job. For many people in health care professions particularly, AIDS is providing an opportunity to evaluate their motives and skills to do rigorous and demanding work. In looking at our motive and vocation, we find a way to work through our fears and frustrations. If health care professionals cannot find a balance, they might need to reconsider their careers and career goals.

Breaking Isolation

No profession is immune from the profoundly existential questions posed by the child with HIV infection, the employee who has AIDS, the legal and political implications of sound public health, and the battle against hysteria and homophobia. Even those counselors or clergy who have given their lives to serving those with AIDS must constantly review where they are. Counselors working with people with AIDS must continually question themselves. "Can I take on another client who is showing symptoms? Do I want to end up with a totally AIDS-affected client population?"

Sometimes counselors will despair and get angry as they lose friends and clients. The author recently spoke to a man in his late 30s, involved most of his life in human services, who was now caring for a man with AIDS in his own home. Painfully he told of how he moved into his new home several months earlier. "I had to move house on my own with no one to assist me because all of my friends are gone now." There is something profoundly tragic about a 30-year-old man left friendless because those close to him have died of AIDS. The same "abandoned" look could be seen on the face of 70- and 80-year-olds in warehouse-like geriatric homes in Ireland. All their contemporaries had gone and they were merely waiting their turn to die. Counselors can learn much form the collective experience of seniors who have lost spouses after many years of relationship. As the extended family disintegrates in cities all across the Western world and an ageist culture does all it can to deny aging, there is an amazing resource in the elderly, neighbors, family, or members of religious congregations who *know* what many people affected by AIDS are going through.

Friedman's "family model" can be helpful to clergy and counselors seeking to build a support system for their clients and themselves. The family model has been a great resource in the parish of All Saints Church in Pasadena, California. Some of the greatest supporters of AIDS work at All Saints Church are a group called "Senior Saints" who get together for a potluck each week. The unfortunate ghettoization of gay versus straight and young versus old can often be healed in places like a religious congregation. The parish church or synagogue may be the *only* place left in society where this intergenerational diversity can take place. Without this connection to a community of seniors, children, expectant mothers and others, where life and death are both embraced and expressed, counseling would be meaningless. This integration is life-giving to all involved. For people with AIDS, the grieving, and the worried well, this represents a "whole" community in which healing, communication, support and dying well can take place.

An Emerging Family Consciousness

It was only 60 years ago that millions of people in Western Europe were wiped out by a great flu epidemic. That painful collective consciousness is still alive in those who remember and in the legacy of community response. For example, in 1933 the author's grandmother gave birth to his father and named him after a 14-year-old boy who died in that epidemic. The boy's mother had helped with the author's father's birth at a time long before maternity wards existed. When the author was born, he was given the same name as his father.

The legacy of community response still exists today, though perhaps under the surface. Counselors have only to ask or reflect, and in doing so can discover a community consciousness and collective expressions of loss and grief. In every village in Ireland and England memorials have been erected with names of young men in their late teens and 20s who were killed in the battlefields of France during what is euphemistically called the "Great War." Even those who did not live in America during the Vietnam War weep at the Vietnam Memorial with its half-emerged list of names in black granite. Looking a certain way at those lists of names one can see one's own reflection in the painful memorial—its half-covered position in the Washington earth reflecting American consciousness over a tragedy that is still not fully owned or grieved.

In 1988, most cities in the United States contributed panels of cloth, like quilts, that carried the names and personal stories of people who had died from AIDS. These panels were often made by lovers, friends, and family members. The Names Project Quilt is a significant contribution to the struggle with community consciousness: It is a way of grieving and sacramentalizing (offering an outward visible sign of an inward spiritual experience) the AIDS crisis. This was profoundly felt during the 1988 Episcopal Church's General Convention in Detroit that coincided with a 2-day visit of the Quilt. Some of the members of the board of the National Episcopal AIDS Coalition had worked hard to ensure a booth at the convention that would educate, advocate, and develop compassion in our congregations. There was excellent media coverage and nine excellent AIDS-related resolutions passed both legislative houses. However, it was a simple ceremony of dedicating three new Episcopal AIDS panels to add to the existing 44,000 panels that really touched people deeply. Midwesterners, WASPS, bishops and a cross-section of the American public were visibly moved by what they saw on the stony quiet floor of the Convention Center. Many editorials and after-convention reviews reflected the impact the AIDS quilt seemed to have made, burning itself into the very hearts of a significant section of the community that will never be the same. The presiding bishop, Edmund Browning, was heard to say privately after the ceremony, "This is the most significant thing I have done here." The quilt is a modern day cairn.

In Los Angeles, in the past 3 years, community consciousness has been helped through the organization of 10 specific liturgies called "AIDS masses." These masses encompass a Eucharist with an AIDS-related homily, special prayers and readings for healing and courage, and a remembrance of those who have died. They occur almost every 3 months in parishes all over the diocese with eight being celebrated by the bishop of the diocese. The local Catholic archbishop also presided at an AIDS mass and was visibly affected by a 3,000 strong congregation of mainly gay Catholics and their friends. The AIDS masses also recognize significant individuals in local communities who have shown personal leadership and courage in medical, spiritual, educational, and political strategies in dealing with AIDS. The masses help people to grieve, to center themselves in the important community values of care, compassion, and solidarity, and to offer to God the people they love, miss, and hurt for, as well as their own fears. In the beginning when AIDS was still highly stigmatized (the days before Rock Hudson was diagnosed) the masses attracted massive media attention. To have a bishop saying mass in a church for AIDS was controversial and highly political. In those parishes that had the courage to sponsor an AIDS mass, there has been a renewed commitment to the ministry of healing of the church in caring for the sick, their families, and caregivers. There is also a new dialogue between the church and the gay and lesbian community. In retrospect, the AIDS masses' most significant contribution has been the renewal of commitment by several key parishes in Los Angeles Diocese to minister to and with gay and lesbian people. More significant, and perhaps surprising, is that many of the heterosexual parish members *wanted* to be involved in this ministry.

AIDS at the Parish Level

In All Saints in Pasadena, California, the AIDS Mass in 1986 led to the creation of the All Saints AIDS Service Center that is currently the principal AIDS-related mental health and case management project for California's Western San Gabriel Valley, employing 12 full-time staff and 250 volunteers. The parish community of the past 20 years has greatly contributed to various social health and peace and justice issues, so working with AIDS was seen as a natural profession of a concern for the welfare of the local community and advocating for the oppressed while healing the sick. All Saints staff has been careful not to develop AIDS programs that are overtly religious or exclude people on religious grounds, with the AIDS-affected community largely unchurched and largely damaged by religious and secular homophobia.

There are several parish programs other than the AIDS program that meet the spiritual needs of the client population. People are encouraged to integrate into programs like Bible studies, discussion groups, and worship services rather than to duplicate them. Gay and lesbian people are welcomed at this parish and an active gay and lesbian support group [Gays and Lesbians All Saints (GALAS)] has been providing spiritual and social programs for the last 3 years. It has been important to separate the issue of homosexuality from the issue of AIDS ministry. The AIDS ministry has been successful because the parish community is already aware and working on its homophobia and is committed to diversity within the congregation. Inservice training programs for staff and informational programs on gay and lesbian people as well as active participation and leadership of gay and lesbian people have helped raise consciousness in the congregation. It would be impossible to provide the trust and honesty needed for a strong and safe pastoral and community relationship with a gay person with AIDS without a congregation working through its homophobia and issues around sexuality and diversity. Congregations that are largely White and homogeneous are usually unlikely to welcome gay people or minorities and may patronize or proselytize persons with AIDS or the worried well. The various "change ministries" like Exodus International and some Catholic attempts at ministry to the gay community have deep philosophical and theological problems with honestly nurturing gay and lesbian people. Heterosexual members of the All Saints Staff are reminded that every time a gay man or woman comes to church, he or she is coming back to the place where they first heard that their "love is not good" and that they themselves were unlovable.

Religious homophobia is a frighteningly destructive phenomenon that often kills people spiritually and sometimes even leads to physical death. For example, one of the author's closest friends, Frank, who died from AIDS, confessed from his darkest self-loathing as a gay man that he wanted to die from AIDS. Somewhere inside his heart he had picked up a wrong message about himself that he carried with him most of his life. In the last 2 weeks of his life, while hospitalized, he was surrounded by so much love and affirmation from his friends and family that he could no longer believe bad things about himself. He died loving himself for the first time and was fortunate to have had 2 weeks to do a deep spiritual self-reappraisal.

Many religious institutions, particularly the fundamentalist wing of the church, inadvertently destroy and maim people through homophobia. It is often forgotten that the crucifiers of Jesus and the murderers of the prophets were deeply devout religious people who wanted to maintain the status quo and thought they were doing God's will. The same forces are still at work in deeply devout, well meaning people who maintain that AIDS is somehow a manifestation of God's punishment on a sexually promiscuous society or chemically addictive people.

AIDS patients and their families and friends will encounter prejudicial attitudes at some level as they interact with society. This will often stimulate early memories in individuals of a damaged self-image, usually influenced by parents, peers, religious people, teachers, and others in leadership positions. These reactions can be the window through which those early memories can be healed with the client integrating more positive values and self-image into his or her contemporary situation. Spence (1986) outlined some personal and group exercises for integration of adult reality with the negative tapes first heard as small children. One of the exercises involves two people facing each other. The listener holds the other person in complete respect and positive regard without any form of criticism or negativity. As the other person recalls painful or disempowering situations, emotions of inadequacy, failure, a lack of skill, intelligence, sexual attraction, a sense of isolation, or withdrawal of love and support may emerge. As adults we can look at the old hurts and, with the partner's help, own our true sense of goodness and self-worth as they tell us what they see. The process of recognizing the inherent worth of a human being fraught with negativity is illustrated in the following case example.

In the summer of 1988, one of the board members at All Saints who is a person with AIDS was in the hospital for the amputation of his right leg. The day following the amputation, he was in great pain and needed medication. In the midst of all this a homophobic religious nurse told him she hoped he knew that God loved him because AIDS had obviously resulted from his gay life style that was against God's will. She did not say "AIDS is a punishment from God for your gayness," but it was certainly communicated that he was living immorally and punishment for self-destructive behavior was inevitable. Armando was very gracious to her, took the opportunity to give her some AIDS and theological education, and made a formal complaint to the hospital. The effect of all this on his spirit, however, was enormous. He was from a Catholic Hispanic background and the nurse stirred up all of his negative self-image issues. The next day, Armando had requested anointing with holy oil and the laying on of hands, a traditional Christian symbol for healing and love. Six of his closest friends and the author used this opportunity to surround Armando symbolically with the reality of his goodness as a gay man and the reality that he was incredibly loved by those present and by God. We stood around his bed acknowledging that what happened to him was painful and emotionally draining. We affirmed what we loved about him. Many of his friends spontaneously shared their love for him with humor and deep emotion, during which he closed his eyes, relaxed, and breathed deeply. We used guided imagery of "a healing sphere of light" entering his body and his heart. We also touched him and anointed him with the holy oil. We all participated in the experience. As a priest I was supported in my ministering to Armando by a community of his friends. Armando smiled deeply and shared how loved he felt. Within 3 weeks he was out of the hospital and made a remarkable recovery from his surgery.

The love and reality of healthy relationships penetrate the deep dark places of self-loathing and self-hatred. This can be facilitated by community experiences like the one described. At the AIDS Service Center one of the 10 support groups specializes in guided imagery, meditation, acupressure, massage, and touching. This seems to be an important therapeutic support system for some of the clients and staff. It operates in conjunction with more traditional psychosocial programs, many of them facilitated by a mental health professional. On a weekly basis there is a small intimate worship group that celebrates the Eucharist together and ends with the "laying on of hands." This is a traditional demonstration of solidarity with the sick or suffering where a priest or group of worshipers lay their hands on the head, shoulders, or body of a person who is seeking some form of comfort, healing, or release from pain or anxiety. The physical touching is usually accompanied by an oral prayer on behalf of the person for healing. This traditional liturgical form has proven to be a therapeutic approach for some of the AIDS-affected population.

More contemporary "alternative" or "new age" therapies also have been successfully utilized by the AIDS-affected community. However, some patterns have emerged and some philosophical or theological areas should be avoided. Some "new age" theories include the idea that sickness is caused by a subconscious decision to sabotage or not to accept "health" as the rightful human experience. This translates into the notion that "I can choose if I want to be sick or healthy. If I have AIDS and am sick, it must be my fault. I must have done something wrong or I am just not meditating or believing in myself enough. If I want these problems to go away I have control and responsibility for it all." Death is also seen as a conscious choice where people "leave the planet" (to use a new-age euphemism) after completing their spiritual work in the body. The danger with this approach is that it can end up reinforcing denial in the AIDS-affected community or making individuals feel that hey have completely failed in life and health.

There are three positive aspects to healthy spirituality that can be integrated with modern psychological approaches to healing. First, communities most oppressed or marginalized can heal negative self-images through the positive reinforcement of their love, integrity, worth, talent and spirituality. Initially, healers often have to *exaggerate* the reality of oppressed people's goodness and lovableness so that it finally penetrates and overpowers the negative messages they learned as children. This can often be structured in group work or in individual counseling sessions.

Secondly, touching is healing. There is an almost universal feeling of being dirty or untouchable that many people with HIV feel. Being touched by another—a holding of hands or hug or more liturgical forms of touching—are all necessary for spiritual and emotional healing and growth in this crisis. When healers do not know the ailing person very well, it is often helpful to them to ask permission to hold or touch them. Close friends can hold too, particularly when someone feels "untouchable" or "unlovable." It can also be healing just to be held while talking or crying. Physical demonstrations of caring and loving can counter the oppression and negative energies people with AIDS feel. Although this may sound strange to some therapists, it has been this author's experience in working with people with AIDS that expressing intimacy physically is very important. Many local AIDS organizations train volunteers in massage and other forms of physical contact with persons with AIDS. This is an important service to people who, as a group, are often isolated and left untouched by society's fear of contagion.

Developing People's Innate Spirituality

It took 2 years at the AIDS Service Center to help clients relax around the spiritual aspects of AIDS. This is partly a reaction by gay men to their homophobic experience of traditional churches and the subsequent denial of their inherent spirituality. Churches have traditionally portrayed gay people as immoral and sinful and have greatly misused biblical quotations like the Sodom and Gomorrah story to denounce homosexuality. Some churches have refused membership and ordination to gay people, and many gay people still regard the church as the source of most of society's homophobia and prejudice against them (see Boswell, 1980). Monica Furlong (1970) sees a direct link between this suffering and spirituality. She writes in her book, *Traveling In*:

> The people whom I have loved best have all known some experience akin to this. One of them stammered, two experienced severe maternal deprivation, two were homosexual, one was seriously rejected and bullied by his peers. What made them special was not the original wound, but the fact that it seemed to open a door, which in others remained closed, a door which led into a landscape of joy. This does not happen automatically as a result of injury—people can be injured, yet remain unaware—but I know of no one who seems able to talk of this landscape without having know the pain first. (p. 29)

John Fortunato's excellent book, *AIDS–The Spiritual Dilemma* (1987) further develops a theological and pragmatic approach for gay and lesbian people. He states that the gay community's spiritual wealth has to be shared at this time with their heterosexual brothers and sisters, particularly to help them process a more honest and appropriate theology of sexuality, sensuality, love, and death. AIDS will finally help the gay community and others get over their sophisticated "denial" around death.

> Most everyone would agree that it could not have come at a worse time. Here we had almost succeeded in obliterating death from our consciousness. We had

worked so hard for so long. More than a century of
progressively hiding the Grim Reaper, or euphemizing
death, of phoneying up corpses, of putting fake grass
around the hole and leaving before the box was lowered. And we were within a hair's breath of our goal.
(p. 93)

There is a direct connection between this "suffering community" and spiritual formation and development. Articulating
these experiences of "exile" and "calling" is important if spiritual people are to somehow make sense of their lives and loss.
This experience, when articulated through writing, poetry, and
art, can break down the denial and externalize the pain, grief,
anger, and suffering associated with AIDS. Creativity in general
may be the key to the question, "How do we survive multiple
loses in our lives?" This articulation is itself profoundly spiritual
and theological, reflecting our journey and moving us along at
the same time. For the past year, the All Saints AIDS Service
Center has been producing a 20–page journal entitled *Asklepios*,
named after the Greek god of healing. It is a window to the
AIDS experience for its 2,000 readers each month. It has helped
people share their stories, articulate their varied experiences,
and show solidarity with one another as a caring community as
seen in the following excerpts:

YOU'VE HELPED US COPE

*Contributed by Joe Goodwin, a member of the AIDS
support group.*
My wife and I were caregivers for our son, John,
during his fight with the AIDS virus and all of the
opportunistic diseases to which he was susceptible. All
Saints AIDS Service Center provided us with a lot of
information. We found that listening to other PWAs'
experiences with drugs and medical treatment made
it much easier for us to participate with our son and
his medical team. It made us knowledgeable enough
to the point where the medical team used us to determine reactions to medication; we kept track of time,
amounts, nausea, diarrhea, fever spikes, and mental
state. In return, the medical team kept us informed
on PCP, MAI, various fungal problems, and KS, plus
the purpose of tests and the validity of test results.

We've used information we received from so many
people at AS/ASC to fight fevers, stop diarrhea, whet
our son's appetite, and do a lot of practical things that
helped John's quality of life that we don't remember
whom to personally thank. All we can say is we love
you all. But there was a lot more than the practical
things that we acquired from AS/ASC; it had to do
with our emotional states. Some of the emotional problems were not directly connected to AIDS, but were a
by-product. How does an adult who has been finan-
cially devastated cope with returning to live with his
parents? How do the parents cope with the emotions
of the returning adult son? What we, and I mean the
whole family, found was that discussing these problems
at AS/ASC group meetings somehow led us to an acceptance that made it a lot easier to cope when all
parties had been able to get to the root reasons for the
anger, frustration, and feelings of losing control. We
don't mean the problems were solved; it's just that we
learned to cope with them. It wasn't unusual to come
to the group an emotional mess and leave feeling like
that 600-pound gorilla was off our back.

The result of our relationship with AS/ASC has
been that the last months of John's life were filled with
beautiful moments that the family will always cherish.
If left on our own we never would have progressed in
time through the initial trauma stages to arrive at acceptance and to have enjoyed so much the time we
had together. If our son hadn't had AIDS and we all
had been able to live lives of the normal span of years,
we wouldn't have known each other any better or loved
each other more than we do now. This brings us to
another aspect of our relationship with AS/ASC; we
want to pass on to other caretakers and PWAs the
message that when AIDS enters a family the experience isn't all bad. What seems to be required is to work
through the problems as quickly as possible and enjoy
your new, deeper relationship with your loved one.

JUNE 22, 1988

Last night I dreamed
    about telling my father I have ARC.

I was scared, as I usually am
     in my recurrent "I'm dying of AIDS" dreams.
Upon waking up, I slowly remembered
     that I don't have AIDS.
I'm not even HIV-positive (I don't think).

So why do I have these nightmares?
What am I afraid of?
I'm one of the lucky ones.
Aren't I?
But . . .

Will I die of old age, impoverished and alone?
Will I be tortured, raped, or murdered?
Will my life be snuffed out in a car crash?
Will I get cancer? ALS? Muscular dystrophy?

I've always "known" I'm going to die.
But I never really believed it
     until my friends came down with AIDS.
Is it comforting to know what you're going to die of?
The unknowns about my own dying are beginning
     to terrify me.

—Lee Rowen

Dixieland

"Well, I wish I was in Dixie,"
isn't that a song?
"Look away, look away,"
same song?
". . . and die in Dixie,"
wrong tune.

You died in your bed
with flannel sheets and
six pillows.
With a black down comforter
and blue pajama tops.
You were propped up
like the little boy who died
in a book of bible stories
my pediatrician had in her office.

You had morphine going into your veins
and tortured, ragged breaths

leaving your body.
You had a raging fever
that glistened as beads of sweat
on your forehead.
You had my tears splashing on your hand
and your fingers failed to grasp mine in return.

I died in your bed
with flannel sheets and
six pillows.
With a black down comforter
and tears that lodged in my throat
no matter how furiously they flowed.

"Old times there are not forgotten,"
still that song?
"Look away, look away, look away . . ."
Well, let's finish it–
"Dixieland."

—*Melinda A. Welch*

Homecoming

Dedicated to my son John
January 1956–April 1988

Son you have come home.
You are not seeking promises,
all you want is my love.

You know well
what I have deep in my heart,
only love and my labor for you.

You need my hands,
my weariness, that you may rest,
and a love that can continue to love.

Son, you have looked into my eyes.
Smiling, you pronounce my name.
You shall find peace
amidst those who eagerly wait.

I have left you to go into the sky.
Now I am lost in my cry.
I am your mother, your friend.

Your love will last forever,
your faithfulness is as permanent as heaven.
With you at my side
I shall seek another day.

—*Carmen Goodwin*

Encouraging people to write about what they are going through
and having it published is a wonderfully powerful way for the
AIDS-affected community to reflect and experience their calling. It counters the tremendously debilitating feelings of powerlessness that people with HIV infection feel.

Making People Feel Clean and Loved Through Traditional Symbols

Feelings of being "dirty" that often link disease, sexuality,
and racism are inherently spiritual in nature. Dr. William Countryman's book *Dirt, Greed and Sex* (1988) links sexuality and
disease with the biblical concept of "purity." AIDS is a purity
issue. These concepts are spiritual and theological and cannot
be tackled only on an intellectual or behavioral plane. The Jewish and Christian scriptures attest to the importance of healthy
eating, drinking, sexual, and social practices that were either
ritualized or were developed into laws. The Jewish laws ritualized good dietary practices of a people intent on survival. Those
who did not follow these laws were "unclean" or "dirty" and
were to be avoided outside the tribe or society. These attitudes
profoundly influenced Christianity, which still regards creation
as inherently sinful, fallen, and dirty. Baptism with water is the
ritual that symbolically makes people "clean" and "good."

Touching and symbolically washing can be helpful antidotes to this debilitating stigma. Many people with AIDS have
been baptized as Christians, and a theological understanding
of this "rite of initiation" could be a great source of healing and
empowerment. The more traditional usage of blessing oneself
with holy water on entering or leaving a church or a blessing
of a liturgical gathering with holy water is also a physical manifestation of cleanliness as God's people. On Maundy Thursday
there is the symbolic representation of love and servanthood at
the traditional washing of feet, enacting Jesus' washing of his
disciples' feet. The author knows of no greater symbol of intimacy apart from sexual intercourse that describes love and

nurturing than washing, anointing, and massaging someone's feet, as the following personal example illustrates:

> When Frank was dying in London, both of us found it difficult to share our feelings about what was happening. I wanted to celebrate the Eucharist with him—liturgically sharing the broken bread and cup of wine, symbolizing the feast and the experience of suffering. I wanted a symbol or vehicle to express our connectedness and love. Frank wasn't particularly religious and it was, therefore, not appropriate for us to do the Eucharist together. In the middle of a pedicure, however, I reached for some oil and began to massage his feet, which he thoroughly enjoyed. Between the words and polite talk something more profound was expressed. He *knew* what I was doing. It was a sort of preparation for burial, a "safe" symbol, a moment of intimacy as friend and priest. It was an important part of our rituals of closure and celebration of our lives together. The action was more powerful than anything we might have spoken. Later, we would use other symbols to say goodbye. In his final conscious moments Frank was unable to speak because of the life support system. Through a "speaker board" he pointed to letters that spelled out "I loved rediscovering you and I always will." The power of those letters, those symbols, are with me forever.

Helping people use their symbols and traditions at moments when words seem inappropriate is a wonderful gift. It can facilitate healing at our deepest level and can express our common solidarity. It is the author's belief that this is the greatest contribution the religious and spiritual community brings to the AIDS crisis.

As AIDS moves into the Hispanic and Black communities, the spiritual dimension of AIDS will only be heightened. These two historically oppressed communities have found solace and empowerment from Christianity, which ironically was also used to oppress them. The model described for the gay community of working through its negative self-image, self-oppression, and self-destructive behaviors can be applied to these communities. There are obvious sexual stigmas and fixed attitudes, particularly to homosexuality, that need to be worked through in both communities. Working with families and church-extended fam-

ilies may be easier in these communities where family values
are still strong and the extended family still seems intact. Research done to set up an All Saints Spanish-speaking support
group found that a woman psychologist or priest provided the
most accepted and comfortable leadership for this group. The
woman or priest is seen as a nurturer and protector of the
vulnerable. Here again, spiritual values and metaphors will help
counselors and clergy integrate AIDS within communities who
are having a difficult time with prevention and education. The
religious community, particularly the Black gospel churches
and the Roman Catholic and charismatic churches in the Hispanic tradition have a major role to play in preventing the
spread of the disease and organizing the local community to
care for the sick and grieving. Professional relationships with
clergy and leading laity by psychologists and others engaged in
AIDS ministry should be of the highest priority as they prepare
for future changes in the AIDS-affected population. Most cities
in the United States have active AIDS interfaith councils or task
forces that can provide many resources at a local level and often
a great deal of "moral clout" when it comes to defeating unhealthy legislation, mobilizing a community for particular projects, or promoting AIDS awareness programs. Ironically, the
religious community often holds the keys to both future problems and future solutions in any community. The Roman Catholic Church could be the most powerful institution in the United
States for AIDS prevention (particularly among Hispanics) if it
advocated the use of condoms for prevention of AIDS. The
church, in calling for a moral consciousness and compassion
for people who are ill, has done more than any community
organization in pushing mental health care providers, politicians, and the general public into the more acceptable "inte-
grationist" position for persons with AIDS rather than the
isolationist position.

It will be important for counselors to try to understand the
part played by spiritual formation in the lives of their clients.
For many gay people, the church, a common vehicle for spiritual formation, has been hostile and a bastion of oppression.
In rejecting the church, many gay people feel alienated or without a "family" or reference point. Those who go into "new age"
religions can often reinforce those earlier spiritual images of
guilt and failure, or instead can break into new levels of consciousness with improved self-esteem, self-worth, and social
integration.

In the "life and death" situation of AIDS, profound questions force all people involved to look for meaning and points of reference in their experiences and be more introspective and reflective. A healthy spirituality can help people through difficult decision-making processes, and a spiritual support group can give people social support and intimacy at a time when they may feel terribly inadequate, frightened, and alone.

Conclusion

During the last 4 years of full-time AIDS ministry, the author has worked with the patients, families, congregations, minorities, health care providers, psychologists, clergy, business leaders, politicians, and the man and woman in the street. Maintaining his sanity and sense of meaning in this "warlike holocaust world" has required deeply personal, spiritual "well-drilling," or suffering the consequences. In these 4 years the author has been closely associated with spiritual people and has constantly used them as a sounding board for his own reflections, anger, and insights as he sought to interpret and integrate these experiences into his own life. This has recently been formalized through a monthly weekend support group of three people, all involved with AIDS-related work and members of All Saints parish going on retreat outside of Los Angeles. There they eat, laugh, cry, share Eucharist, write journals, read, and renew and love each other through some moments to themselves. This support system has been an invaluable spiritual source and breaks the sense of isolation that many feel.

Each counselor who commits to the "long haul" will need to develop safe spaces for him- or herself, carved out of the pain and tragedy and sheer neediness of the AIDS crisis. It will be at places like this that they will be able to share their deepest fears, move beyond their own inner limitations, and be nurtured through the crisis. Through AIDS-related support groups and parish congregations, counselors can attempt to create an intergenerational diverse family to absorb some of the pain of AIDS. In doing so, counselors will help to integrate rather than isolate.

References

Boswell, J. (1980). *Christianity, social tolerance and homosexuality*. Chicago: University of Chicago Press.

Countryman, W. (1988). *Dirt, greed and sex*. Philadelphia: Fortress Press.

Cotter, J. (1987). *The cairns network*. Exeter: Cairns Publications.

Fortunato, J. (1987). *AIDS: The spiritual dilemma*. San Francisco: Harper & Row.

Friedman, E. (1987). *Generation to generation*. New York: Guilford Press.

Furlong, M. (1970). *Traveling in*. London: Hodder and Stoughton.

Section Four

THE PROFESSIONAL CHALLENGES FOR COUNSELORS

Section Introduction

The issues raised by the AIDS crisis are not confined to people infected with the HIV. Counselors, too, have had issues thrust upon them by the AIDS crisis. This section examines professional challenges to counselors doing AIDS work.

One of the biggest questions counselors face is how they can help to reduce the continual spread of AIDS. In chapter 12 on education and prevention, Garfield and Hammond write that "if counselors wish to assist in preventing the spread of AIDS, education is the only weapon in the prevention arsenal." Chapter 12 underscores how important it is that all counselors be educators. The chapter proposes specific techniques for effective AIDS prevention and education programs.

In chapter 13, Green tackles one of the more difficult areas in the counseling profession: legal and ethical issues. From his unique position as a psychiatrist and lawyer, Green describes the dilemma AIDS poses and the duty to warn potential victims. His chapter clearly and concisely provides counselors with information they need to face the difficult decisions of conscience, statutory law, and ethical guidelines.

No Longer Immune: A Counselor's Guide to AIDS concludes with chapter 14 by Namir and Sherman, which is devoted to countertransference issues. Counseling people with AIDS is an experience unlike any others most counselors have had. Namir and Sherman write that whether a counselor's experiences "are seen as stressors, leading ultimately to 'burnout' or as opportunities for both personal and professional growth," will often depend on the counselor's awareness of countertransference issues. The authors of this chapter discuss countertransference from an expanded view, referring to a counselor's conscious and unconscious emotional reactions to clients and the nature of the HIV spectrum diseases. The authors examine situational

and therapist factors in countertransference and give suggestions for confronting countertransference issues and preventing burnout. Namir and Sherman conclude their chapter, and
the book, with an honest, sensitive, and revealing look at the
countertransference issues they themselves experienced during
their early work with people with AIDS.

Counselors must open their hearts and help those affected
by the AIDS crisis. Counselors cannot avoid their responsibility
to educate, to work toward the prevention of the spread of
AIDS. Counselors cannot escape the legal and ethical questions
of working with people with AIDS. Finally, and perhaps most
importantly, counselors cannot ignore the toll that doing AIDS
work takes on them personally. AIDS brings with it great opportunities for counselor growth and development, countered
by situations of depletion and despair as well. Counselors must
find, for themselves, sources of both inner and outer support
in order to truly embrace the notion that they are, in the face
of the AIDS crisis, no longer immune.

Chapter 12

AIDS EDUCATION AND PREVENTION

Nancy J. Garfield and Rev. James Hammond

Counselors and human development specialists are in an excellent position to assist in slowing the spread of AIDS. They have not only the ability but also the access necessary to provide education and information about the human immunodeficiency virus (HIV), how it is spread, and how one can reduce his or her risks of exposure. If counselors wish to assist in preventing the spread of AIDS, education is the only weapon in the prevention arsenal—there are no vaccines, there are no antidotes, there are no cures, and there are no quick fixes.

AIDS education and prevention programs are being developed nationwide. The first programs were targeted for the gay community, and were successful in achieving a reduction of high-risk behaviors because of their audience-specificity. Primary health education programs are most successful when they have a circumscribed population with training that addresses their particular needs. Becker and Joseph (1988) found that risk reduction has occurred more often by the modification of sexual or drug-use behavior than its elimination. Longitudinal descriptions of individual behavior demonstrate considerable instability or recidivism. Fineberg (1988) indicated that although "some striking changes in behavior have occurred, especially in homosexual populations in areas with high prevalence of AIDS, educational efforts to date have succeeded more in raising awareness and knowledge about AIDS than in producing sufficient changes in behavior." Sorenson, Gibson, Heitzmann, Dumontet, and Acampora (1988) developed a prevention program for drug abusers in a residential treatment program.

The preliminary results of the 6-month follow-up show that their program increased participants' (N = 56) knowledge about AIDS and changed some attitudes that had put them at risk of acquiring or transmitting the HIV infection.

Agreement has not been reached on the content that composes adequate AIDS education because of various moral or ethical postures from which sexuality is approached; agreement has not been reached on the methodology of AIDS education in part because each educator must adapt her or his style to the task to be effective. In this chapter, a framework is presented upon which specific educational programs for AIDS prevention may be developed. This framework is based on the belief that essential elements of style or procedure must be incorporated in any AIDS education presentation, whoever the audience may be.

Themes in Successful AIDS Education

The topic of AIDS is highly charged emotionally, and it is of particular import that when presenting an educational program, counselors attend to the themes identified in this section. Both authors are trained and experienced AIDS educators, and both strongly believe that the guidelines set forth in this chapter will enable any interested person to maximize his or her ability to be effective as a communicator.

AIDS Education Should Be Appropriate

Each audience is different in important ways, some obvious, others subtle. Astute educators will be able to assess these apparent differences quickly, and be able to tailor the message to fit the receivers. For example, the educator's vocabulary needs to be modified when speaking with third graders rather than adults. Audiences composed primarily of clergy will be more interested in pastoral issues whereas audiences composed primarily of nurses will be more interested in issues of hands-on care. Some differences are less apparent though equally important. The authors of this chapter failed to recognize one such element when hosting a workshop for ordained ministers. The workshop was labeled in our community as a "liberal" event; conservative ministers did not register in large numbers.

Because our goal was to help prevent the spread of AIDS by educating ministers, and not to change the perspective from which they approached AIDS, we erred in letting our bias affect the outcome of our effort.

AIDS Education Needs to Be Accurate

AIDS is a relatively new disease that has an exceptionally high morbidity rate. Most people who contract the HIV virus will eventually fall victim to the disease. In light of the facts about AIDS, to say that AIDS is an overwhelming disease is to grossly understate the case. In one recent educational event, the male partner of a monogamous, *heterosexual* relationship of more than 20-years standing shared with those assembled that his intimate encounters with his spouse were suffering from all of the news about AIDS. Irrational as it may be, people are simply scared to death; unfounded as it may be, people are reacting in their lives, often inappropriately, based on their fears. In 1988, national attention was given to two extremes of opinion about the safety of heterosexual relationships, one published in *Cosmopolitan* stating that "there is almost no danger of contracting AIDS through ordinary sexual intercourse" (Gould, 1988, p. 146), the other in a book by Masters, Johnson, and Kolodny declaring that AIDS infections are "running rampant" in the heterosexual community (1988). Neither extreme represents the best information available, and neither is helpful in the battle against the spread of AIDS. Information being taught must be accurate; to the extent that the public becomes distrustful of information being disseminated, to that extent the public will ignore the same. Counselors have a wonderful opportunity, seldom enjoyed, to address an audience hungry to learn. Audiences must be assured, however, that what they are hearing they can trust with their lives. Instead of dismissing the potential for the spread of AIDS through oral sex as unlikely, responsible counselors and educators will be better advised, and their clients and audiences better served, to respond more truthfully to such a question: "We do not believe that AIDS is transmittable through oral sex, we have no documented cases of such transmission to date, but we simply do not know for sure; always use a condom or a dental dam." (A dental dam is a piece of latex or similar material available in varying sizes from dental supply houses and recommended for use as a protective barrier during cunnilingus and oral-anal sex.)

Some audiences will come with preconceived notions about the disease that are based on beliefs and not on facts. One example that surfaced in an event being hosted by the authors was a gentleman who stood to share with the assembled his belief that AIDS is God's punishment upon a "perverted segment of the population," and that the disease has only coincidentally spread to others. Such a belief puts an impediment in the educator's path of disseminating accurate information in a simple and straightforward fashion. No amount of logic will dislodge such a belief in many cases, so the educator is left with only one option—finding a way to work the message around the bias. "Although I may not agree with your conclusion, I hope you will agree with me that we need to use condoms if we are to prevent a further spread of this disease." To attempt to fight the battle on the grounds of someone else's belief is a mistake. It is better to take each person where he or she is and provide the most up-to-date and accurate information you can.

AIDS Education Needs to Be Articulate

The educator should assess the audience to know to whom he or she is speaking and make decisions about how much and what kind of information is to be presented. The temptation to speak on epidemiology is almost overwhelming in an AIDS presentation because such information is so informative, but it is highly inappropriate in a gathering of third graders. Third graders need to know much more basic information—what AIDS is, how AIDS is spread, what the body parts are and how each is involved, what body fluids are and which are most risky, what touching is as well as what kinds of touching are o.k. and what kinds are not o.k., whether they are at immediate risk of getting AIDS, and so forth. On the other hand, a gathering of physicians will need to know the epidemiological information, along with all of the above! Educators need to be articulate with their information. They need to operate under the assumption that their audience has limited knowledge about AIDS and its transmission. In any audience there will be people present with varying degrees of knowledge about AIDS. For example, many physicians believe that documentation of HIV status in a medical record or chart will help to prevent members of the medical community from contracting the disease. The educational fact is that all patients ought to be treated with universal blood and body fluid precautions by all medical personnel at all times; when such precautions are taken, charting HIV status is rendered moot.

AIDS Education Needs to Be Accessible

Statements like, "This is the fourth time I've been to a seminar on AIDS, but it is the first time I've really understood that I am not at risk for AIDS by hugging someone," heard time and time again by AIDS educators, demonstrate that the messages that need to be disseminated about AIDS require more than one exposure to be learned. Information that has highly charged emotional content or import, such as the potential for dying, is often more difficult to learn. Anyone attempting AIDS education must be aware that multiple exposures are necessary for most people to learn accurate information about AIDS. There are several ways that you can encourage people to further their exposure to the information. Seminars can be planned to meet over three 2-hour sessions rather than one 6-hour session; bibliographies and other appropriate printed material can be provided to participants in educational events, free of charge if possible; sign-up lists can be arranged so that lists of people in attendance as well as lists of resources and speakers can be circulated. Networking is one way to increase the amount of exposure to the information available about AIDS. The counselor and educator not only need to provide information, they must first overcome fear, and, having provided information, motivate behavior change. Multiple exposure to the information often is required if a counselor or educator is to accomplish all three tasks.

AIDS Education Must Be Affordable

"I would have come to your gathering but I simply could not afford to take the time off from work. Even if I could have taken off from work, $75 is far more money than I have for such an event." Those are the actual words a colleague spoke to one of the authors when she was asked about the potential for carpooling to an AIDS educational event sponsored by one of the leading medical institutions in the country. When hosting an event, difficult decisions must be made about cost versus availability. No one wishes to lose money by hosting an event, yet many people who wish to learn cannot pay. Tapping federal, state, and municipal resources is one way to work around the problem of how much to charge for an educational event. Frequently private sector resources are available to assist, not only in planning an event, but also in carrying it out. Local AIDS education groups often can provide experienced speakers without fee. Many churches and schools can tap such resources without paying. If the goal is to reach as many people as possible with information about preventing the spread of AIDS, dollars need not be a hindrance to attendance. Many people have more investment in educational endeavors for which they have to pay something, so at least a minimal fee for any event, perhaps stated as a "materials cost," is recommended.

AIDS Education Should Be Amoral

Counselors come to educational opportunities with their own values, their own ideas about right and wrong, good and evil; many counselors and educators have clear ideas about what is moral and what is immoral. Providers of information about AIDS are no exception because AIDS tends to strike at disadvantaged groups of people, many of whom are often disenfranchised. Consider for a moment that homosexuals, bisexuals, substance abusers, and infants are among those most likely to develop AIDS. If counselors and educators approach their efforts through the eyes of one moral perspective, they stand to lose whatever influence they may have with everyone who holds a differing moral stance. Instead of offering controversial opinions, educators need to center on a subject that can be agreed upon, for example, that information about AIDS needs to be disseminated.

AIDS Education Should Be Affective

"The audience was hushed as he spoke. Tears filled the eyes of many; it was a moving experience. John, a PWA, a person with AIDS, had just shared his story, and clearly many in attendance were caught up by the emotion of the moment—some perhaps even changed their outlook on PWAs because of John's willingness to share." Educators working in the field of AIDS for any length of time over the past several years have no doubt been privileged to participate in an event such as the one described above—the moving appearance of a PWA to tell his or her story to an audience of generally mixed sympathy. One such PWA even spoke eloquently to his audience, telling those gathered they did not need to protect him or his feelings as they asked him questions. "I'm a big boy," he told his tentative audience, "I can take it." As moving as those talks may be, how many educational events *require* the presence of a PWA? There is a difference between featuring a speaker because he or she has something to add, and simply mollifying voyeuristic inclinations. The added benefit that comes to an AIDS presentation by providing a vicarious experience of the disease is highly questionable except under the most unusual and demanding of audiences. It is almost always costly to a PWA to make a personal appearance, and although it may be loving on his or her part, how loving is it to him or her?

Instead, educators can help to make their own presentations affective by teaching people to keep sex erotic and exciting! Many men and women seem to believe that sex can no longer be fun if they must be responsible, if they must plan, and if they must use a condom or a dental dam. Counselors and educators can teach people that safer sex practices can actually heighten their lovemaking experience. Teasingly, the partner can offer to assist in placing a condom; affectionately, more touching can be added to the script; caringly, the couple can simply become more conscious of new ways to please. Paying attention to safer sex (condoms, dental dams, and spermicides) can be presented as truly loving behavior.

An equally important part of amorous AIDS education is the openness and accessibility of the presentors to all in attendance. It is important to recognize that persons in your audience will need to be able to question you, to approach you for clarification, perhaps even to get to know you. You are asking many in your audience to change life views as well as behavior; if you are to be successful, you must be available. That kind of personal availability comes only through a willingness to reach out and love others through your educational endeavors.

AIDS Education Should Be Anecdotal

Although it is generally not necessary to have a person with AIDS in attendance at an educational event, it is important to personalize the event for those participating, to make it real.

One way to personalize the data is to invite people whose lives have been touched by AIDS, from hands-on caregivers to parents and relatives of PWAs. One most impressive presentation was the mother of a person with AIDS speaking to a group of clergy. She told of a minister refusing to make a house call on her dying son, and of another who did visit, only to give the son a lecture on sin. Professionals experienced the insensitivity of their beliefs by being brought face to face with their behavior. The more the lives of people can be touched, the more the message gets through. Slide shows are great, videos are superb, but neither is a substitute for first-hand reporting from people actually involved—one presence is worth a thousand words!

AIDS Education Should Be Apologetic

Apologetics in the theological sense means the making of a reasoned defense on intellectual grounds for one's beliefs. AIDS educators must be trained, willing, and desirous of being apologists for AIDS education. Many people simply don't want even to hear about AIDS; they will resist with every ounce of their being learning what they need to know for their own health and well-being. Some grudgingly assert that AIDS education is important, but only for others—the ones likely to become infected. AIDS educators and counselors need to lobby at every opportunity with officials at every level for the presentation of effective programs. If counselors and educators go to a house of worship, they should speak with the leader about an AIDS education program for persons in each age group. If they have children in school they should speak to the administration about the need for teachers to be trained and equipped to do AIDS education in the classroom. Counselors and educators can make appointments with the elected legislators in their district and impress upon them the need not only for programs but also for funding. Write letters; send telegrams; make phone calls; take people to lunch.

AIDS Education Should Be Astonishing

Few topics that challenge the abilities of an educator have as many built-in aids as does AIDS! If one wishes to "hook" an audience, one need only get up and say, "if you don't listen to what I have to say today, your inattention may kill you." One can make use of the startling statistics that this disease presents: 100% of persons with AIDS are likely to die from their disease; infection rates are nearly doubling each year; use of a condom decreases your chance of contracting AIDS on any given occasion by a factor of 10. Any of the above attracts the attention of audiences. Along with the sensational figures, there is some solace and comfort. The number of medical personnel who have seroconverted due to inadvertent needle-sticks is remarkably well below one half of 1%—good news not only for persons employed in the medical field, but for all. (This low seroconversion rate supports other data suggesting that AIDS is hard to get, even when one is inadvertently inoculated with infected fluid or tissue.) There is no evidence to suggest that casual contact vectors AIDS—people won't get it from living in the same house with a PWA. Mosquitoes do not spread HIV. Whether the educator snags his or her audience with the good news or with the more sensational news, the point is simple—the disease AIDS is filled with opportunities to assist the educator to do the job. Use eye-catching data to drive home the message; rely upon the high levels of affect generated by the material to motivate audiences. Structure your educational event to maximize the advantages inherent to the materials you are trying to teach. For example, if you want to wake your audience up, take out a condom, blow it up, pass it around, put it over your head, do whatever it takes to help people remember your message: Condoms are to be used!

AIDS Education Should Be Authentic

The key to authenticity is in the speaker. Even the most truthful data will go unbelieved by an audience that does not trust the presentor. Therefore, counselors and educators must find a way quickly and effectively to gain their audience's respect if they wish life-changing behavior to result from their presentations. Showing vulnerability is one way to foster people's acceptance and trust. Educators can share stories about how AIDS has affected their life, or how they have intervened in the life of another. One AIDS educator was talking with a young girl and her boyfriend about safer sex when she discovered that the couple's name for his penis was "Freddy." To explain the importance of using condoms, she said, "Put a hat (condom) on Freddy each time you have sex." Her intervention was effective not only with the young couple in terms they could understand, but also gave her a story to share in future educational events. Cicero said that a good speaker is a good person who speaks well. AIDS educators who are effective will fit his model—they will be good people, genuinely concerned about others, who present their message with authenticity.

AIDS Education Should Be Awesome

Many workshops are filled with too much free time; when professionals attend an educational experience, the presenters need to remember that professionals are for the most part busy people who do not take well to having their time frittered away. Counselors and educators cannot hurt themselves or their workshops by overscheduling; the worst thing that can happen is that the workshops will run a bit late. Plan a variety of presentations to keep people from becoming bored. If you, as educator and presenter, take your message seriously, the chances are that those in attendance will as well, whether they agree with you or not. Extemporaneous remarks offered by even well-informed persons do not receive the kind of favorable feedback that a thoroughly prepared presentation does. A higher level of learning is required to attain the goal of motivating people to action in the prevention of the spread of HIV. It is one thing merely to teach, another altogether to motivate!

Methodologies for Presentations

In this section specific suggestions about methodologies, as well as some potential pitfalls in preparing an AIDS education program are discussed. Each educator should adapt the material that follows for best use in his or her presentation.

AIDS Educators Need to Use All Available Media

Some of the most successful methods of conveying to an audience the pain inflicted by AIDS can be found in several high-quality videotapes. No one wishes to attend a workshop only to be placed in front of a television all day, but one or two carefully chosen tapes of modest length can do wonders for getting a difficult message across. It is necessary to measure the audience and choose such tapes with care, and to pay attention to dated material as new findings and new statistics obtain, but when tapes of high quality are used with care by the educator, the results can be very gratifying indeed. In addition to the video medium, audiotapes, books, pamphlets, slides, overhead gels, and printed handouts can help make a workshop successful. If the educator does some basic research ahead of time, he or she will discover far more material available than can possibly be used in any given presentation. Sources to tap are our local and state health departments, private community agencies devoted to AIDS, libraries, hospitals (especially teaching hospitals), and in some communities, churches. Some denominations have excellent educational packages designed for group work already prepared for educators wishing to work with smaller numbers of people.

AIDS Educators Need to Pay Attention to Techniques of Delivery

Most educators need to be reminded that how something is said can spell the difference between being heard and not being heard, often literally. Is the sound system sufficient for the crowd? Can the slides be seen? Are there enough televisions so that everyone present can see and hear the selection of videotapes? Why work so hard to stage an educational gathering and then fail to meet the audience's human needs to be able to see, to hear, and to take notes? Counselors have a great deal to offer as educators about the need for the prevention of the spread of AIDS; they should be prepared to try to do all in their power to accomplish the goal. The cost of failing to get the message across is high, unacceptably high, if the reason is the failure to pay attention to simple details.

Educators May Benefit From Working in Small Groups

The benefits from working in smaller groups of people are already well documented and well known to most educators and counselors—more people become more involved, each person is heard, individuals' questions can be addressed, resistance to process is easier to deal with, and so forth. Working with small groups, however, does require prepared personnel; with

a little advance preparation facilitators can help in AIDS presentations even if they are not thoroughly knowledgeable about
AIDS. The successful small group experience will be an open-
ended one that gives each participant a chance to voice his or
her own opinion while also learning about others'. Experience
has proved that it is always best to give some rudimentary facts
prior to sending people into small groups to grapple with hard
questions. Small group work is best midway in a workshop, after
participants have had a chance to come on board with the topic
but well before wrap-up, so that issues generated in the small
groups can be shared and discussed. Educators who wish to use
the small group format need to plan what happens so that
control of the event is not lost. This can be done through proper
staffing and proper tasking. Small groups have the immense
advantage of personalizing the educational experience, but the
disadvantage of being time-consuming.

AIDS Education Benefits From Experiential Techniques

People learn best by doing, not by looking, observing, and
listening. If a presentation about AIDS is given to a group of
counselors, it is well to have participants practice counseling
techniques. If a presentation is given to a group of teachers,
have the teachers get up and teach for a time something they've
learned. If the proper use of condoms is being taught, do a
"hands-on" presentation where the condoms are distributed,
the packages opened, and the contents felt and observed first-
hand. One of the authors was disturbed to watch a nurse give
a demonstration on HIV prevention techniques in the work
place, be it hospital or doctor's office, that included the drawing
of blood without the recapping of needles. The nurse asked
for a volunteer so that she could demonstrate the techniques
she was recommending, then proceeded to draw the "victim's"
blood without the approved standard procedure of wearing
rubber gloves! Her message was lost because she failed to practice what she was teaching. People learn by doing; providing
opportunities for them to do so helps them learn.

AIDS Educators Must Not Be Bashful About Repetition

Research has demonstrated that people need to be exposed
to information about AIDS on several occasions before the mes-

sage begins to take. Most educators will have only one opportunity to address any given group, so it is necessary to present the same data from several perspectives. It is worth the risk of being called a repetitive speaker if the audience remembers what was presented. If educators tell the audience, "AIDS is preventable," as they begin the workshop, as they come back from a lunch break, and several times just before they leave, some people may be angry, but "AIDS is preventable" will be on the tips of their tongues and forged in their minds. If people remember that AIDS is preventable they will know enough to find the answers they need. Repetition is the key to teaching that "AIDS is preventable!"

Pitfalls To Avoid in AIDS Education

It is important to identify clearly any roadblocks that might obstruct the goal of preventing the spread of AIDS through effective educational programs. The following should be considered as potential problems.

Jargon as an Enemy to Effective AIDS Education

The first concern is the use of jargon, especially in heterogeneous audiences. If counselors are speaking to an audience full of MDs they can easily infer that most will at least understand the terms, but many lay people will trip over HIV, ARC, AZT, antibody, PWA, FWA, and even perhaps such terms as "seropositive." How many people in an average audience will understand that AIDS is an acronym, standing for the formal name of the syndrome—acquired immunodeficiency syndrome? Although the technical term is condom, some people use the word "rubber" whereas others prefer prophylactic or sheath; youngsters, particularly, are often confused by the multiplicity of terms and are not always certain just what is being talked about unless counselors and educators overcome their embarrassment and make themselves crystal clear. With all audiences, but especially with young people, the more formal terminology should be used when discussing the sexual aspects of the spread of AIDS. A meeting of the minds needs to be held early on to ensure that all understand the terms you are using. One excellent icebreaker for gatherings of young people is taking the time to list all of the various words they use for genitals. Unless counselors are clear to the audience, they may not know what is being talked about and the message will be lost.

Question Your Assumptions

"Physicians will be well informed about AIDS." "People have seen a condom and know how to put a condom on an erect penis." "The average monogamous couple's sex life is unaffected by AIDS." These assumptions and others like these are not necessarily correct and can cripple a presentation for two reasons: first, inaccurate assumptions can keep counselors and educators from presenting vital information that people may need to know in order to understand AIDS prevention; second, assumptions can keep counselors and educators from hearing what others are saying. By way of example, presenters at a gathering where AIDS information was being presented to a large number of heterosexuals, most of whom live in monogamous relationships, centered their program on the sexual vectors of AIDS; in doing so they missed an opportunity to uncover significant pain in the lives of some people in attendance who felt they were at risk for HIV infection due to other vectors (transfusions, blood splatters, and sexual relationships with intravenous drug users). AIDS educators should not make any assumptions.

Avoid Statistical Boredom in AIDS Education

Although AIDS is a source of interesting data, there is a danger in presenting too many statistics. For each statistic to be presented, educators should assess whether their audience needs to know this fact. Some audiences will need to know facts—by way of example, medical personnel can benefit from learning about the low seroconversion rate from needle sticks, mentioned earlier. Most audiences, however, do not gain from the presentation of statistics and may actually be hurt. At one presentation where the audience was given epidemiological data on the prevalence of HIV infection rates by state, some in attendance commented that "We don't have a problem here in Kansas, so we don't have to worry about precautions." The presentation of statistics gave participants the misleading notion that AIDS exists only in New York City or in San Francisco. In reality AIDS exists in every state in the country. It is a mistake to present too much statistical data in AIDS education events because such data are often boring and sometimes downright misleading. Data should be used only on a "need to know" basis.

Pay Attention to Audience Reticence in AIDS Education

Although giant strides have been made over the past generation in opening communication among people on issues sexual, many people are still uncomfortable talking about "private" issues in public. Some people even feel repelled when formal medical terminology is used, never themselves finding the need to use the words "anus," "vagina,"or "penis." AIDS education counselors and educators must find ways to make talk about matters sexual commonplace, to look for ways to help people feel comfortable talking about things heretofore often unmentioned. It takes all of the interpersonal skills that counselors and educators can muster to find ways to open the avenues of conversation, to enable people to talk about subjects for years considered forbidden in polite society.

What They Need to Know

When we talk about providing AIDS education we are really discussing how to help people prevent themselves from becoming infected with the HIV virus and learn the facts about the course of the infection.There is some basic information that needs to be included in every AIDS/HIV educational program. The data change so rapidly that it will be important to contact local AIDS support agencies, the county or state health department, or the Centers for Disease Control to obtain the most current statistical and medical information. The *MMWR*, (*Morbidity and Mortality Weekly Report*), provides updates on health guidelines and recommendations for programs such as the "Guidelines for Effective School Health Education To Prevent the Spread of AIDS." *The Journal of the American Medical Association* and *The New England Journal of Medicine* contain the most current research articles about AIDS and HIV infection.

People attending AIDS programs need to know that the routes of HIV transmission are blood and body fluids (primarily semen and vaginal secretions). At-risk behaviors are sharing intravenous needles and paraphernalia, and having unpro- tected sex. Sadly, babies born to a mother who is HIV-positive are also at risk. Many people are afraid that AIDS is transmitted by touching and hugging, sharing kitchen utensils, or being in the presence of someone known to be HIV-positive. AIDS is not transmitted through such *casual contact*.

When talking about safer sex, counselors and educators should include the following advice. The way to be safest is to be abstinent. If abstinence is not an option people wish to choose, they should avoid high-risk behaviors such as having sex with multiple partners, or with people who have or have had sex with multiple partners. During intercourse, condoms contain- ing a spermicide with nonoxynol-9 should be used. Research seems to indicate that the spermicide nonoxynol-9 further re- duces the risk of contracting the HIV. Practices that may injure body tissues, for example anal sex or rough vaginal sex, should be avoided. Oral-genital contact should be avoided unless the man is wearing a condom or a dental dam is used. Although many caution about open-mouthed, intimate kissing, recent re- search (Fox, Wolff, Yeh, Atkinson, & Baum, 1988) seems to indicate that this is less of a risk than first thought.

Counselors and educators can suggest that there are many ways to be intimate and to be safe in addition to protected intercourse. Mutual masturbation can enable partners to reach orgasm and be less at risk if they avoid sharing of semen or vaginal secretions. Social kissing and body massage, frotage (the rubbing of bodies together), and hugging are other ways to increase intimacy. Most important, counselors can encourage their audience or client to talk with their partners about sex and intimacy and explore what is arousing, and what new safe ways they can find to enjoy being together.

People need to be taught about how to use condoms. In addition to the information provided here, there are several books about condoms that are useful (Breitman, Knutson, & Reed, 1987; Everett & Glanze, 1987). Only latex condoms should be used because the natural condoms are not uniform in thick- ness. A condom is to be unrolled onto an erect penis prior to any contact with the genitalia of the partner. It should be un- rolled all the way to the base of the penis, allowing 1/4 to 1/2 inch at the tip or end for ejaculate. After the man ejaculates he should hold on to the condom and pull out while the penis is still hard. The condom should be discarded in a way that no one will be in contact with the semen. A new condom should be used each time one has sex. Petroleum-based lubricants, such as petroleum jelly, should not be used; such lubricants can cause premature deterioration of a condom. Condoms should not be stored for a long time in a wallet or purse because they may develop little holes. (Several companies are now selling hard cases in which to carry condoms, the use of which may alleviate the problem.) Condoms should not be left in places of extreme heat such as a glove compartment. The expiration date on the box of condoms should be checked when purchasing them because they become less reliable as they age. Condoms with non-oxynol-9 are preferable and additional nonoxynol-9 spermicide should be used in the condom.

Safer sex for women in lesbian relationships includes protection from blood (including menstrual blood) and cervical and vaginal secretions. Cunnilingus is risky unless one is sure her partner is not HIV-positive, so the use of dental dams is recommended.

People attending education programs will want to know if they have placed themselves at risk in the past. They will want to know about "the HIV antibody test." The test was designed to assess the safety of the blood supply for transfusion practices. It indicates if there are HIV antibodies in the blood, not if someone has AIDS. The test is not 100% accurate. A small percentage of the time the test gives falsely positive or negative results (Myer & Pauker, 1987). The accepted practice is to do a screening test, such as the ELISA (enzyme-linked immunosorbent assay) and, if the results are positive, to do a confirmatory test, most often, the Western Blot. The results of the test provide information about one's antibody status at that particular point in time. The test is most apt to be able to report antibody status at a time of no less than 2 weeks after the at-risk behavior, although it may take as long as 6 months for the test to diagnose a positive antibody status. It is important for counselors and educators to make clear that there is no test, at this time, that will provide immediate information about recent risky behavior.

The question of who should be tested is a difficult decision and has many ramifications. People who have been diagnosed HIV-positive have experienced discrimination that includes loss of job, insurance, and home. Alienation from friends, family, and co-workers also occurs. Before deciding to be tested, persons need to be aware of the possible psychological and social/

legal consequences of the test. The authors discourage the practice of HIV antibody testing unless there is a clearly indicated medical reason for it. An example of a clearly indicated medical reason is establishing the etiology of neurological symptoms such as memory deficits, gait irregularity, psychomotor retardation, and dementia. Although some people believe that everyone should know his or her antibody status, others (including the authors of this chapter) believe that such information gives people permission to be less careful. Whether those concerned are practitioners who come into contact with blood or body fluids on the job, or simply people who wish to use a negative HIV status to avoid safer sex practices in a casual relationship, the scientific reality is that knowledge of HIV status is not a prevention technique or even a prevention factor. The recent development of experimental protocols for the preemptive administration of AZT and other AIDS drugs to persons at high risk makes each individual's decision even more personal. The efficacy of these experimental protocols has yet to be demonstrated, and the associated side effects of such prophylactic treatment can be severe.

The diagnosis of AIDS is made on the basis of a number of clinical symptoms. These illnesses may include, but are not limited to: Kaposi's sarcoma, HIV encephalopathy, histoplasmosis, non-Hodgkin's lymphoma, HIV wasting syndrome or pneumocystis pneumonia. A person may meet the CDC case definition for AIDS and not have a positive HIV test. In providing education and information about AIDS, counselors and educators must be careful not to diagnose or to give that impression. Whenever possible, counselors and educators should have the name and phone number of the AIDS community service organization and the county health department available to share with audiences or clients should they wish further information.

Finally, counselors and educators must be aware that in talking with people about AIDS education and prevention, they must discuss that a diagnosis of HIV-positive or AIDS affects more than the person with the diagnosis: the family and significant others of the infected person will be affected by the diagnosis as well. Both the diagnosed patient and his or her family will experience depression, rage, and other emotions. When educating, counselors must sensitize all to assist those dealing with this horrible illness to provide as much love and support as possible. Only as counselors work together to provide education and support can there be any hope of preventing the spread of AIDS.

References

Becker, M.H., & Joseph, J.G. (1988). AIDS and behavioral change to reduce risk: A review. *American Journal of Public Health, 78,* 394–410.

Breitman, P., Knutson, K., & Reed, P. (1987). *How to persuade your lover to use a condom . . . and why you should.* Rocklin, CA: Prima Publishing and Communications.

Everett, J., & Glanze, W.D. (1987). *The condom book.* New York: Signet.

Fineberg, H.V. (1988). Education to prevent AIDS: Prospects and obstacles. *Science, 239,* 592–596.

Fox, P.C., Wolff, A., Yeh, C., Atkinson, J.C., & Baum, B.J. (1988). Saliva inhibits HIV-1 infectivity. *Journal of the American Dental Association, 116,* 635–637.

Gould, R.E., (1988, January). Reassuring news about AIDS. *Cosmopolitan, 204,* pp. 146–147, 204.

Masters, W., Johnson, V., & Kolodny, R. (1988). *Crisis: Heterosexual behavior in the age of AIDS.* New York: Grove Press.

Meyer, K.B., & Pauker, S.G. (1987). Screening for HIV: Can we afford the false positive rate? *The New England Journal of Medicine, 317,* 238–241.

Sorenson, J.L., Gibson, D.R., Heitzmann, C., Dumontet, R., & Acampora, A. (1988, August). *AIDS prevention with drug abusers in residential treatment: Preliminary results.* Paper presented at the 96th Annual Convention of the American Psychological Association, Atlanta, GA.

Chapter 13

AIDS AND THE DUTY TO WARN: ETHICAL AND LEGAL FACTORS

Richard Green

> *All that may come to my knowledge in the exercise of my profession or in daily commerce with men, which ought not to be spread abroad, I will keep secret.*
>
> Hippocratic Oath

The uniqueness of AIDS, fatal and sexually transmitted, provokes an unprecedented legal and ethical dilemma. Compounding this combustible mix is the additional, incendiary component whereby most persons with the syndrome are members of stigmatized social groups.

The central ethical and legal dilemma facing the health care professional with an HIV-infected patient is best serving the needs of that patient while concurrently serving the needs of others. As the AIDS epidemic escalates, with both cure and prevention seeming remote, public clamor for protection affects the private anguish of the infected. Caught between these poles is the conscientious psychiatrist, psychologist, counselor, or social worker.

Under the common law (laws that evolve from court rulings rather than from legislatures), a person generally owed no duty to control the conduct of another, nor warn those endangered by such action (Restatement 2d Torts; Prosser, 1971). However, an exception to this absence of duty has been carved out where the person stands in some special relationship to either the person who could be controlled or to that person's foreseeable victim (Restatement 2d Torts, §315–320). That the physician, therapist, or counselor does stand in a special relationship with the patient is well established: ". . .a special relationship exists between the actor [therapist] and the third person [patient] which imposes a duty upon the actor to control the third person's conduct" (Restatement Section 315 (a)). With this principle as backdrop, the stage is set for major ethical and legal issues that confront the professional whose patient has AIDS. The dilemma pits the tradition of patient confidentiality against the hazard to a nonpatient.

Case Law

Although it is popularly believed that information communicated by a patient to a physician has always been confidential (or privileged), such protection is a relatively recent legal development. Despite the Hippocratic Oath admonition, there was no prohibition under the common law to communicating medical facts about a patient without the patient's consent. Indeed, it was long after the common law established a legal basis for confidentiality between attorney and client that any statutory provision was established for physician-patient privilege. (A cynical view of this progression is that the common law, promulgated by the legal profession, was concerned more with its professional interests than with those of physicians.) With the advent of psychiatry and other professional services directed toward the amelioration of emotional distress, newer professions sought and achieved comparable patient privilege. Thus today, patients (often called clients) of psychologists and clinical social workers, plus those of marriage and family counselors, may also hold privilege. In California, statutory confidentiality is provided for physicians, psychologists, clinical social workers, and marriage, family, and child counselors (Sections 990–1018, California Evidence Code). The holder of the privilege is the patient. Generally this means that unless the patient agrees to break the confidence, the health care professional may not. Exceptions to this privilege exist, however.

Precedent-setting court cases underscore the professional's responsibility to third parties (persons other than the professional and the patient), despite statute-created privilege. The seminal legal case establishing a psychotherapist's duty to warn, in violation of confidentiality or privilege in California, is *Tarasoff v. Regents of the University of Southern California*. There the court ruled that a therapist has a duty to use reasonable care to warn a foreseeable and identifiable third party against a serious threat of danger by the therapist's patient. "The protective privilege ends where the public peril begins" (17 Cal. 3d 442). The *Tarasoff* court held: "[D]efendent therapists cannot escape liability merely because (the victim) herself was not their patient. When a therapist determines, or pursuant to the standards of his profession should determine, that this patient presents a serious danger of violence to another, he incurs an obligation to use reasonable care to protect the intended victim . . . . The discharge of this duty may require the therapist to . . . warn the intended victim . . . or to take whatever steps are reasonably necessary under the circumstances" (17 Cal. 3d 431).

Tarasoff has been codified in California Evidence Code (CEC) §1024. "There is no privilege . . . if the psychotherapist has reasonable cause to believe that the patient is of such mental or emotional condition as to be dangerous to himself or to the person or property of another and that disclosure of the communication is necessary to prevent the threatened danger." The explanatory comment following this exception to confidentiality states, "Although this exception might inhibit the relationship between the patient and his psychotherapist to a limited extent, it is essential that appropriate action be taken if the psychotherapist becomes convinced during the course of treatment that the patient is a menace to himself or others and the patient refuses to permit the psychotherapist to make the disclosure necessary to prevent the threatened danger" (CEC at 140).

Even before *Tarasoff*, the duty to warn a potential victim in another medical circumstance had a precedent, a circumstance relevant to AIDS. In 1920, in a case involving syphilis, the Supreme Court of Nebraska ruled that the information given to a physician by his patient, though confidential, is given subject to the understanding that, if the patient's disease is found to be dangerous and so highly contagious or infectious that it may be transmitted, the physician may disclose the information to others to prevent the spread of disease (*Simonsen v. Swenson*, 1920). Other, more recent court examples reinforce the physician's liability for both not diagnosing and reporting disease (*Hofmann v. Blackman*, 1970; *Wojcik v. Aluminum Co. of America*, 1959).

A fetus or child, not just an adult, may be a foreseeable victim. Because at least half of all fetuses gestating in an HIV-positive mother are born HIV-positive, this rule is especially salient. The child becomes a "second order" foreseeable victim when its mother is exposed to the virus. California case law has extended liability to the children of "first order" victims. In *Hedlund v. Supreme Court* (1983) a mother sitting with her child was shot by a psychologist's patient. The child, witnessing the attack, allegedly suffered emotional injuries. The court held that the duty the therapist owed to the woman extended to her minor child because the risk of harm to the child was foresee-able—the child was indentifiable as a person who might be injured if the patient attacked the woman.

With specific regard to AIDS, individual case law has been transformed into statutory formality. California law protects the physician who elects to warn. "No physician and surgeon who has ordered a test to detect antibodies to the probable causative agent of acquired immunodeficiency syndrome and who has the results of the test shall be held criminally or civilly liable for disclosing to a person believed to be the spouse of a patient that the patient has tested positive . . . ." (Deering Health and Safety Code, 1982). Thus no privilege exists regarding disclosure to a spouse. However, spouses, under all state laws, must be of the opposite sex. What of a steady same-sex sexual partner? What of a nonspouse, live-in opposite-sex partner? Or other, more casual partners at risk?

Patients themselves may disclose their HIV status to the state. Then, the state may contact a sex or drug partner: ". . . (a) any person receiving a test for the presence of antibodies to immunodeficiency virus (HIV) may disclose the identity of any sexual partners . . . to the county health officer . . . (c) The county health officer may alert the sexual partners . . . about their exposure, without disclosing any identifying information about the individual making the disclosure . . . ." The same rule applies to those who share the use of hypodermic needles (California Health and Safety Code West, 1988).

What if the physician does not warn? California Civil Code (West, 1988) holds that a psychologist or psychiatrist is not liable for *failing* to warn or protect a victim from a patient's behavior except "where the patient has communicated to the psychotherapist a serious threat of physical violence against a reasonably identifiable victim or victims." Thus the professional must determine what constitutes a "serious threat." Does such a threat include the stated intention by the patient to continue sexual intercourse with an identified partner? And what of the patient with rapidly changing partners?

To keep the AIDS dilemma in perspective, we should note that pyschotherapist-patient privilege is not absolute, even in situations involving medical risk to others. If a patient sues a therapist for malpractice, privilege is lost (California Evidence Code §1004). In insanity or competency hearings, privilege is compromised (CEC §1004). If the psychotherapist is sought to aid in the commission of a crime or tort [a private or civil wrong, other than breach of contract, for which the court will provide a remedy in the form of an action for damages (Black's Law Dictionary, 1979)], there is no privilege (CEC §997).

Professional Societies

Health care societies have also set HIV reporting guidelines. The American Medical Association (AMA), in issuing its ethical guidelines (AMA, 1987), stated that confidentiality is "absolute" until it "infringe(s) in a material way on the safety of another. . . . Those who are not infected . . . are entitled to protection. . . ." Responding to its perception of public health needs and the role of confidentiality, the AMA stated that "[a] sound epidemiologic understanding . . . requires the reporting [on an anonymous or confidential basis to public health authorities] . . . of those who are confirmed as testing positive. . . ." The AMA addressed physicians practicing in jurisdictions where reporting is not mandatory. "The physician should attempt to persuade the infected individual to refrain (from risk activities). . .when persuasion fails, authorities should be notified. . . ." In the event that the physician knows of a specific potential victim, the AMA asserts "a physician may have a common-law duty to warn . . . ."

On the other hand, the AMA (1987) acknowledges that notifications may be prohibited by statute. In that case the AMA endorses legislation that both provides a method of warning unsuspecting sexual partners, and protects physicians from liability for failure to warn. It also establishes standards for informing public health authorities and presents guidelines for authorities when they trace unsuspecting sexual partners. The AMA has called for legislation that would grant immunity to physicians who either notify third parties or choose not to, because the risk is deemed by them to be inconsequential. Disclosure is permissible " . . . with the reasonable belief that . . . the information will avoid or minimize an imminent danger to the health or safety of the patient or any other individual . . . when released . . . to health care personnel . . . in order to assist the patient or to protect the health of others closely associated with the patient." Furthermore, the physician may disclose "after counseling the infected individual to consent to the disclosure to the spouse or other sexual partner . . . . (Then) the attending physician may elect to notify the spouse or other sexual partner of the infected individual. A cause of action will not arise from any such notification. (On the other hand), there shall be no duty on the part of the attending physician or other health care provider to notify the spouse or other sexual partner of an infected individual, (when the physician deems the risk inconsequential) and a cause of action will not arise from any failure to make such notification."

The AMA provisions straddle the horns of the physician's dilemma. When the physician believes that the partner should be warned, the physician is protected. However, when no warning is given, because the physician does not diagnose the risk, the AMA position is similar to current California law. The physician would remain protected. A successful malpractice action for negligence in failing to diagnose might follow, however.

Infected physicians have also been addressed in AMA guidelines. The sick physician is directed not to engage in patient care that creates a risk. If a risk does exist, disclosure of the physician's seropositivity to patients is deemed insufficient; the physician must cease risk contact. However, if the physician poses no risk, disclosure is not warranted. Prior to the physician making that determination, however, the AMA recommends that the afflicted physician disclose the seropositive status to colleagues for their consideration of any risk posed.

The American Psychiatric Association (APA) has also issued guidelines on confidentiality. "Psychiatrists should not discuss their patients' care, (but) in cases involving imminent danger to others, psychiatrists must balance their duty to protect patients' confidences against their responsibility to members of the public at risk" (APA, 1987).

The APA policy statement stresses that " . . . any breach of confidentiality should be a last resort . . . . " Recognizing that

APA policy may conflict with law, guidelines suggest that "where conflict exists, attempts should be made to modify laws in accordance with the principles expressed herein."

At the onset of a psychiatric evaluation, according to the APA, when suspecting that a patient is HIV-positive or is engaging in behavior that is known to transmit HIV, the psychiatrist should inform the patient of the limits of confidentiality (a psychiatric "Miranda" warning). When the psychiatrist deems that there is a risk to third parties, the psychiatrist should first advise and work with the patient "either to obtain agreement to terminate (the) behavior . . . or to (agree to) notify identifiable individuals who may be at continuing risk . . . ." If the patient rejects this agreement, "it is ethically permissible for the physician to notify an identifiable person whom the physician believes to be in danger . . . ." (APA, 1988).

The APA also issued interim guidelines on handling HIV infection in outpatient services. HIV testing should be performed on a case-by-case basis with informed consent when medically indicated. The responsible psychiatrist should disclose the information (about HIV infection) to appropriate staff only after discussions with the patient, when the psychiatrist determines that appropriate treatment of the patient requires such disclosure. If a patient known to be HIV-infected engages, or threatens to engage, in behavior that is known to transmit HIV disease, the psychiatrist shall assure that, in addition to education, appropriate clinical steps are taken to attempt to modify the behavior (APA, 1988, October 7).

When should physicians recommend or request that a patient be tested for exposure to HIV? The California Board of Medical Quality Assurance in its guideline issues in August, 1988, urged that seven categories of patients "should be routinely counseled about and tested" for HIV. These include men who have had sex with men, hemophiliacs, persons seeking treatment for sexually transmitted diseases, persons with a history of intravenous drug use, women of childbearing age and having identifiable risks for HIV infection, prostitutes, and persons from geographic areas where heterosexual transmission of HIV is common. Physicians should also consider HIV testing with persons undergoing evaluation for clinical signs and symptoms compatible with HIV infection, and for persons who received blood components or transfusions between 1978 and 1985. Thus, the physician who plays ostrich and does not encourage testing may be vulnerable to violation of professional guidelines. However, whether a patient falls into one of these seven categories may not be readily apparent.

The APA has addressed the problem of unidentifiable third parties who may be at risk, that is the transient sexual or drug partner of a patient. "It is ethically permissible for a physician to report to the appropriate public health agency the names of patients (who are) HIV-infected and whom the physician has good reason to believe are engaging in behavior which places others at risk. . . ."

Discussion

Thus, professional conduct, to be safe, is defined by these statutes and guidelines. But professional conduct, to satisfy the professional's concerns for ethical conduct at variance with statutes or guidelines, may pose a personal dilemma. Statutes and guidelines can, at times, be compromised in spirit, if not in letter. But professionals who flaunt the law or their professional society guidelines risk legal sanction or loss of licensure.

In mandating the reporting of high-risk behavior, the duty to warn may be counterproductive, however. Psychotherapists and counselors cannot deal with matters unknown to them. A basic psychiatric principle is that "every person, however well motivated, has to overcome resistances to therapeutic exploration. These resistances seek support from every possible source and the possibility of disclosure would easily be employed in the service of resistance" (Goldstein & Katz, 1962). As another forensic behavioral scientist noted, "It is clearly recognized that the very practice of psychiatry vitally depends upon the reputation in the community that the psychiatrist will not tell" (Slovenko, 1960).

Moreover, the historical alienation between psychiatrists and homosexuals is an additional dimension of concern here. Psychiatry led the public perception of homosexuality as a mental disease, and was, for decades, dedicated to the cure of the homosexual's affliction (Bayer, 1981). Many psychiatrists remain convinced that homosexuality is an illness. Thus, the profession has hardly established itself as a trusted ally among the gay community. The majority of homosexuals, not motivated to reorient to heterosexuality, have historically not consulted psychiatrists. The likelihood is remote, then, that they would seek contact under a system in which their potentially most damaging personal revelation was not confidential. Consequently, the highest risk group in the United States for which reporting could be expected to protect others have entrenched biases against communicating with those professionals who are in a position to protect others.

Issues of AIDS reporting are distinguishable clinically and socially from other sexually transmitted diseases (STDs) in which reporting has been held to be the responsibility of the patient or physician. Traditional STDs were not generally identified with stigmatized minority groups. Although the diagnosis of syphilis, and later gonorrhea, carried stigma during a period in which premarital sexual abstinence and marital monogamy were expected, the stigma that attached to violation of these standards was not as substantial as the historic opprobrium attached to homosexuality and intravenous drug abuse. Nor were the heterosexual sexually active singled out for blame for the spread of a fatal disease.

With consequences of AIDS infection higher than those with syphilis in the pre-antibiotic era (many infected persons were spontaneously cured, and those whose disease was progressive did not die for about 20 years) (Clark & Danbolt, 1955), infection with the AIDS virus may be uniformly fatal. Thus there is greater risk of stigma to the infected person when that person is publicly identified, but there is also greater medical risk to the uninfected person if their risk vulnerability is not communicated.

Recent court rulings regarding liability for spreading a sexually transmittable disease have relevance for the communication of AIDS. A New York court ruled that a woman could seek compensatory and punitive damages from her former husband for his alleged transmission of genital herpes. The court held that the husband had an affirmative legal duty to disclose to his wife. Furthermore, the sexual partners need not be married for responsibility to attach. In 1984, the California Supreme Court held that a woman can maintain an action for "damages for severe injury to (her) body, which allegedly occurred because of (the man's) misrepresentation that he was disease-free" (*Kathleen K. v. Robert B.*, 1984). Infection by the AIDS virus, instead of the genital herpes virus, does not seem distinguishable for instituting legal action.

Should therapists require that their patients be tested if the therapist believes the patient to be of a high-risk group and engaging in high-risk behavior? A major damage award may await the psychiatrist who fails to predict a patient's dangerousness from contagion. A 1.4 million dollar judgment was upheld by the highest court of Delaware after it was held that a psychiatrist should have foreseen with medical certainty that a former patient would commit a dangerous act (*Venkataramana Naidu v. Ann D. Laird*, 1987).

Involuntary AIDS testing has precedent. In September 1988, in California, the governor signed a bill allowing courts to determine when a person *charged* (not convicted) with sexual assault may be ordered to undergo HIV testing when the alleged victim so requests (Sexual Assault Bill, SB 2643, 1988). California's Proposition 96, passed by voters in 1988, extends testing because of the alleged victim's fears of transmission via sweat and saliva, and not only blood and semen.

California is not alone in requiring AIDS testing in some circumstances. Illinois has an involuntary or nondisclosed AIDS testing program. There, physicians may test their patients without the patient's knowledge. Although opposed by the Illinois Department of Public Health, and the Chicago Health Department, it was supported by the Illinois State Medical Society.

Thus, the trend is toward limited or no confidentiality for HIV-positive patients. Beyond, what is hoped, the passing scope of the AIDS epidemic, will this shift undermine a major feature of the traditional doctor-patient relationship? Will the medical profession, once held in the highest public esteem, and in recent past eroded by the epidemic of malpractice suits, be compromised further by erosion of the confidential nature of the patient-physician relationship? With the security (perhaps mistakenly, to an extent) held by patients that they could consult a physician for disease or a psychotherapist or counselor for an emotional problem with the assurance of confidentiality gone, helping professions may never regain their position of the highest confidence and respect. These factors play major roles in both the prevention and amelioration of disease, whether the effect be called placebo, faith healing, or positive transference. If so, AIDS may not only destroy many persons, young and old, male and female, of diverse life styles, but its ultimate victim may be an essential ingredient of the health care system itself. Health care workers must face difficult decisions of conscience, as well as statutory law and the oxymoronic phrase "ethical guidelines," as they attempt to serve both their patients and the larger society.

References

American Medical Association Council on Ethical and Judicial Affairs. (1977, reprinted 1987). *Journal of the American Medical Association*, *259*, 1360–1361.

American Psychiatric Association. (1987). Guidelines on confidentiality. *American Journal of Psychiatry*, *144*, 1522–1526.

American Psychiatric Association. (1988). AIDS policy: Confidentiality and disclosure. *American Journal of Psychiatry*, *145*, 541.

American Psychiatric Association. (1988, October 7). *Psychiatric News*, p. 12.

Bayer, R. (1981). *Homosexuality and American psychiatry*. New York: Basic Books.

Black's Law Dictionary. (1979). St. Paul, MN: West Publishing.

California Board of Medical Quality Assurance. (1988, August). *Guidelines*. Sacramento, CA: Author.

California Civil Code Section 43.92 (West, 1988).

California Evidence Code (CEC) §990–1018., 1024.

California Health and Safety Code Section 199.27, 43.91 (West, 1988).

California Voters, Proposition 96, November 1988.

Clark, E., & Danbolt, N. (1955). The Oslo study of the natural history of untreated syphilis. *Journal of Chronic Diseases*, *2*, 311.

Deering, Health and Safety Code of the State of California (1982), §199.27.

Goldstein, J., & Katz, J. (1962). Psychiatrist-patient privilege: The GAP proposal and the Connecticut Satute, 36 Conn. Bar J. 175, 179.

Hedlund v. Supreme Court, 34 Cali. 3d 695 (1983).

Hofmann v. Blackman, 241 So. 2d 752. (Fla. 1970).

Kathleen K. v. Robert B. 150 Cal. App. 3d 992; 997 (1984).

Prosser, Law of Torts. 4th ed. 1971. §56, p. 341.

Restatement 2d Torts. §314–315. Com. c.

Sexual Assault Bill, California SB 2643 (1988).

Simonsen v. Swenson, 177 N.W. 831 (Neb. 1920).

Slovenko, R. (1960). Psychiatry and a second look at the medical privilege. 6 Wayne L. Rev. 175, 188.

Tarassof v. Regents of the University of California 17 Cal. 3d 425 (1976).

Venkataramana Naidu v. Ann D. Laird. Superior Court of the Sate of Delaware, in and for New Castle county: Civil Action No. 79C-JA-97, (1987).

Wojcik v. Aluminum Co. of America, 18 Misc. 2d 740, 183 N.Y.S., 2d 351, 357–58 (1959).

Chapter 14

COPING WITH COUNTERTRANSFERENCE

Sheila Namir and Scott Sherman

Providing counseling or psychotherapy to people who have AIDS involves experiences that may be unique in the therapist's professional life. Whether these are seen as stressors, leading ultimately to "burnout," or as opportunities for both personal and professional growth, will often depend on one's awareness of countertransference issues evoked by working with people who have AIDS.

The concept of countertransference was used by Freud (1910) to refer to the influence of a client on the therapist's unconscious and was seen as a hindrance to effective work unless a therapist overcame it. Since then, the definition of countertransference has been greatly expanded. In 1950, Heimann enlarged the definition of countertransference to include all of the therapist's feelings and reactions toward the client. This "totalistic" view of countertransference (Kernberg, 1965) placed importance on the therapist's countertransference as a tool for his or her work, helping the therapist understand the client's dynamics (see Gorkin, 1987).

The expanded definition of countertransference, and its elaboration by other theorists and clinicians (Cohen, 1952; Little, 1951; Racker, 1957; Weigert, 1954), included an attempt to understand situations that led to the presence of anxiety in the therapist that could interfere with treatment. The potential of countertransference reactions to undermine or assist the therapeutic work is part of the "totalistic" approach.

Cohen (1952) described three broad categories that may contribute to countertransference and anxiety in therapists. These are situational factors, including competence and role issues for the therapist; unresolved neurotic problems of the therapist; and, the overwhelming feelings of the therapist when the client's anxiety is communicated to the therapist.

In this chapter, we will explore countertransference issues that arise in working with people who have AIDS or are positive for the HIV antibody. We will use the term countertransference to refer to the therapist's conscious and unconscious emotional reactions to clients and to the nature of the disease. Following an overview of the literature on countertransference reactions to people with life-threatening illnesses, we will explore issues that confront therapists in working with people with HIV infection or AIDS based on situational variables, therapist factors, and specific client variables. We will then address the common defenses therapists may employ against feelings and reactions aroused by these variables, and suggest ways to confront countertransference issues. By discussing some of these issues, we hope to help therapists recognize responses and feelings toward clients that may contribute to their own feelings of "burnout" or might prevent them from working effectively with people with AIDS.

Overview of the Literature

The literature on countertransference issues specifically with people who have life-threatening illnesses, or are dying, has often focused on whether or not therapists have confronted issues about death in their own lives (Burton, 1962; Clarke, 1981). Explicit in these discussions and studies is the hypothesis that if therapists have confronted these issues in their own lives, they would be better equipped to help others who are dying.

The intense reactions and painful feelings elicited by working with people who are dying are often discussed in books and articles for therapists about working with terminally ill persons (Bascom, 1984; Burton, 1962; Eissler, 1955; Pruyser, 1984; Rando, 1984; Renneker, 1957; Sourkes, 1982; Weisman, 1981). These reactions result from the need for therapists to confront their own separations and losses, fears of illness, death and dying, and unconscious fantasies related to rescuing others from death (Eisendrath & Dunkel, 1979; Sourkes, 1982). An inability or unwillingness to confront any of these reactions can lead to avoidance of clients, overidentification with them, unresolved repetitive grief reactions, or "chronic demoralization" (Pruyser, 1984), and "blaming the victim" (Ryan, 1971) in an attempt to deny or avoid one's own vulnerability or sense of personal failure in rescuing people from illness and death (Renneker, 1957).

In addition to the above, the specific countertransference issues mentioned in the literature include threats to one's sense of power, mastery, and control (Rando, 1984), anger at the dependency needs of medically ill clients (Eisendrath & Dunkel, 1979), over- or underinvolvement, anxiety or depression, and false optimism (Weisman, 1981). We would also include survivor's guilt, subtle homophobia, overvaluing the importance of work with people with AIDS compared to other clients, overestimating or underestimating the seriousness of the disease, and avoidance or denial of discussion topics related to death and dying.

Working With AIDS Clients

The AIDS epidemic in this country has deeply affected counselors and therapists. Few of us have remained untouched by the need to struggle with our countertransference reactions, even if it is on the level of deciding whether or not to work with people who have AIDS. The epidemic has, more specifically, involved us in an existential crisis, a social crisis, and a professional crisis.

The existential crisis relates to our own understanding and beliefs about illness, death and dying, and the intense reactions to witnessing illness and death in so many young people in our country. This can lead to becoming increasingly demoralized, and adopting a tragic view of life. We fight to maintain hope and ward off despair, but the pain of the world is no longer an abstract philosophical idea (Pruyser, 1984).

A social crisis ensues when we become involved in fighting discrimination and negative attitudes toward those who have AIDS; when we become frustrated with legislative and political activities that threaten to harm those we are trying to help; when we confront issues of sexuality, sexual behavior change, and drug abuse; and finally, when we seek to empower disenfranchised members of our society.

The professional crisis may begin with our perceived or actual lack of adequate knowledge and competence in working with medically ill clients. We have to become educated about the complex medical and neuropsychological aspects of AIDS, in addition to the psychosocial aspects of illness, death, and dying. The professional crisis continues when we experience conflicts related to our role as professional counselors or therapists, and the intense demands and needs of people with AIDS. Our training in traditional psychotherapy may become a source of conflict for us as we struggle with the need to be available and responsive, as well as the need to provide support, advice, information, and advocacy for our clients. All of these crises may impede or assist us in our work with people with AIDS, depending on our abilities and willingness to struggle with the countertransference issues they elicit. In his or her work, each therapist needs to determine when unusual behavior and responses to clients may be due to countertransference. We will discuss these in terms of the situational, therapist, and client factors that may contribute to countertransference reactions.

Situational Factors

The nature of the disease is an important source of potential countertransference reactions. One of the hallmarks of AIDS is the relative unpredictability of the course of the illness, which can interfere with a therapist's desire to establish goals, maintain continuity, and feel effective. As a person with AIDS becomes more ill, increasingly physically debilitated, and possibly more depressed, it is more difficult for the therapist to intervene in effective and meaningful ways. Previous treatment goals and interventions may become meaningless or ineffective because of the changing condition of the client. These goals and interventions must be constantly reevaluated based on the client's current physical, emotional, and neuropsychological condition.

Another related issue confronting therapists working with persons with AIDS is the demand of new roles. These roles frequently generate anxiety and insecurity because they often mean that therapists must be in environments with which they are unfamiliar and in which they feel unsafe when compared to their own offices. When a person becomes ill it is quite likely that during the course of the illness he or she will be frequently hospitalized and at times will be too ill to travel to a therapist's office. Therapists who work with clients with AIDS will often have to make hospital visits and home visits in order to continue their work with them. For many therapists, making home visits may feel like an invasion of privacy and a crossing of boundaries. Therapists must be able to explore what internal resistances they have to visiting clients in their homes or in the hospital.

Many people, including therapists, feel uncomfortable in hospital settings because of the preponderance of unfamiliar medical equipment, language, and procedures. Hospitals may also elicit associations with unpleasant experiences. Additionally, visiting a client in the hospital can generate increased anxiety because it is often there that a person with AIDS is the most vulnerable and where the impact of the illness can be seen most clearly. It is important that therapists explore their willingness to make hospital visits, which are time-consuming, and to understand and anticipate the kinds of anxiety and discomfort they may feel in a hospital room.

People with AIDS in therapy often ask medical questions, describe medical procedures and diseases, and ponder the meaning of various laboratory results. For nonmedical mental health professionals, these questions and discussions may generate anxiety as they become aware of their lack of knowledge and competency in these areas.

Therapists must also struggle with the "rules" they have assumed in their practice of psychotherapy. They need to struggle with decisions about giving advice, working with the extended family and friendship network, touching or hugging a client, the fees they charge, and educational interventions. Whether or not the standards of behavior or rules therapists have previously adopted are applicable to their work with people who have AIDS is a source of conflict for some therapists.

Therapists may find themselves in the position of being advocates for clients, as well as speaking and interacting with family members, significant others, and medical personnel. These situations raise issues of confidentiality, and often other ethical dilemmas. The lack of clearly defined confidentiality and ethical guidelines related to people with AIDS is a source of anxiety for therapists. Debates continue in different governmental legislatures, professional organizations, and committees regarding these guidelines or potential laws. A therapist may, however, become obsessed by these arguments, immobilized by the lack of clear guidelines, and fearful of what he or she says or does.

The unpredictable course of the disease, medical crises and treatments, changing treatment goals, interventions, and settings, as well as the demands these place on the therapist for assuming new roles and behaviors are situational variables contributing to countertransference issues. These, however, are intimately connected to therapists' own unresolved issues.

Therapist Factors

Perhaps the most salient issue that therapists working with persons with AIDS must confront is their own mortality. Most individuals do not confront the inevitability of their own death, but rather operate under a system of denial and invulnerability. However, when one works with persons with AIDS, and especially those clients who are near death, it is impossible to maintain one's sense of invulnerability, or to continue to deny the potential of one's own loss and the anxieties that losses often generate. Whenever a client dies, experiences and feelings associated with other losses in the therapist's life come to the fore. The extent to which these previous losses have been understood and resolved will affect the therapeutic relationship with the person who is dying. Every current loss experience necessitates a working through of previous losses and an acceptance of the necessity for allowing for a grief reaction for the person who has just died. The challenge the therapist faces is to confront his or her own feelings of attachment, sadness, anger, and depression related to both previous losses and the current loss.

Therapists place an emphasis on maintaining objectivity and professional distance. These values are stressed in training and in much of what is written about doing psychotherapy. However, therapists do form attachments and bonds with their clients. These feelings of attachment, care, and concern must be acknowledged and validated. Therapists who feel they have been unprofessional in becoming attached and caring for a client with AIDS run the risk of depression and burnout because they may end up feeling alone in their grief reaction. Our sense of our roles as professionals may also make it difficult for us to give ourselves permission to grieve or to participate in rituals that would help us to resolve our grief. The loss of a client often is not defined as an appropriate loss to be grieved, and we may struggle as we attempt to deny these feelings.

An equally important issue for a therapist to confront is, "What is my motivation for wanting to work with someone with AIDS?" Therapists must be clearly aware of what it is that they expect to gain from this work, as well as what is going to be expected of them as they embark on it. Is this a veiled way of working out their own issues of fear of AIDS? Are therapists seeking validation for their own magical thinking that they are immune from exposure to the AIDS virus by exploring how others may have been exposed to it? Is there the hope that they will confront their own fears about death, or work out their own past and potential losses? Is counseling the dying seen as an opportunity for noble, glorious, and profound experiences? One cannot automatically assume that issues of motivation and self-interest will not seep consciously and unconsciously into the therapeutic relationship.

Most of us entered the mental health field because we had a conscious need to help others. Whether or not this was a sublimation of feelings of magical omnipotence may affect our feelings of helplessness in working with people with AIDS. When faced with the barrage of medical symptoms, psychic and physical pain, intense fears and the wish for a cure, we may begin to feel that all our efforts do not make much difference. Our belief in the efficacy of our therapeutic skills, and therefore our therapeutic hope, may be diminished or destroyed.

For many of us, AIDS is not an issue solely in our professional lives, but it is also present in our personal lives. This unremitting focus on AIDS can contribute to feelings of being overwhelmed and overburdened. If we have engaged in behaviors that may place us at risk for having contracted the virus, we may suffer "survivor's guilt," wondering why our clients are ill and not we. If we have not engaged in risk behaviors, there may be an exacerbation of "blaming the victim," attempting to protect ourselves by moralistically attributing blame, thus reducing our capacity for compassion, empathy, and identification, and further stigmatizing people with AIDS.

Our unresolved role conflicts may also create problems in working with people who have AIDS. There may be a tendency to stay within a narrowly defined role, or to focus on professional knowledge and factual or philosophical issues. Ultimately, this is a way to withdraw from people with AIDS. On the other hand, for some of our more isolated clients, we may become their major source of support, leading to conflicts about the limits of our role and responsibilites we can assume.

Client Factors

The most obvious client variables that may contribute to countertransference reactions in therapists are the levels of fear, anxiety, despair, and hopelessness a person with AIDS experiences. We may become overwhelmed if the intensity and levels of any of these reactions are high. Therapists may react differently to clients who are optimistic, who minimize their distress, who avoid talking about having AIDS, or who use frank denial as a defense. It is important that therapists become aware of how these different responses to AIDS on the part of the client may be affecting them and the therapeutic work.

The client's own belief system about life and death may either be in conflict or be congruent with the therapist's belief system. Because of the central nature of these beliefs, the potential for countertransference reactions is strong. A client may seek religious, spiritual, or psychological experiences that the therapist may judge, thus damaging the therapeutic relationship.

Complicating the more general countertransference issues discussed above are difficulties in working with people who have a personality disorder or who may be considered "difficult clients" without the additional burden of being physically ill. Many of us wish to believe that being confronted with a life-threatening illness can help in the development of a positive spirit. We have seen how the crisis has helped some people with AIDS to develop stronger personalities and has given meaning to their lives (Mandel, 1986). These experiences may contribute to problems with those who do not conform to this belief. In fact, a physical illness can exacerbate underlying difficulties in living and coping, and can create profound countertransference issues for therapists (Groves, 1978; Namir & Wellisch, 1985). Groves's discussion of the types of "hateful client" and what they evoke in the therapist is particularly useful. He described four types of difficult clients who are also medically ill: dependent clingers, entitled demanders, manipulative help rejecters, and self-destructive deniers. Clingers evoke aversion, and therapists need to set limits before they become exhausted. Demanders evoke fear in therapists as they attempt to intimidate them through hostility and threats. A countertransference response to demanders may include counterattack. Help rejecters evoke guilt and feelings of inadequacy in the therapist, whereas deniers evoke all of the above negative feelings as well as anxiety on

the part of the therapist because of clients' self-destructive behaviors.

Illness can often cause a regression in people because they
feel more dependent, fearful of abandonment, depressed, pes-
simistic, or angry. An added strain on the therapist may be the
attempt to deny intense and hateful feelings toward the difficult
client. If therapists are to avoid maladaptive solutions to their
countertransference, including unconscious punishment or
avoidance of the client, responding in an empathic way will be
important to determine what is caused by the illness or by fears
and justifiable anger, and what is exacerbated by personality
disorders.

Therapists commonly feel guilty for harboring negative
feelings toward someone who is ill or dying. They do not feel
justified in setting limits or confronting inappropriate and destructive anger. They may internalize the hopelessness and
helplessness that these clients feel (Adler, 1972), making them
ineffective in their work. Attempting to repress the negative
feelings these clients evoke can lead to restlessness, anxiety, and
impatience (Maltsberger & Buie, 1974). It is essential that the
therapist recognize these reactions, and then become able, eventually, to help the client see how his or her behavior affects
other people in ways that make it less likely that they will receive
positive responses. A crucial variable in helping clients with
AIDS to cope and live with their illness will be helping them to
direct their anger in ways that are not self-defeating in order
not to alienate medical personnel and their support networks.

Defenses Resulting From Countertransference Issues

The range of painful and difficult emotions engendered
in the therapist working with someone with AIDS may create
the need for reliance on measures that are protective in the
therapeutic encounter. The most general protective device is
to adhere to a theory about the nature of counseling the dying.
Both empirical research (Lindemann, 1944), as well as clinical
studies (Eissler, 1955, Kübler-Ross, 1969), have led to the development of a number of models that put forth a stage theory
of death and dying. These theories identify stages and processes
that those with terminal illnesses move through. They relate,
as well, to the process of grieving the loss of someone who dies.
Two methods therapists have of protecting themselves from

the range of painful emotions is to rely exclusively on a pre-scribed model of working with a person with AIDS, and to try to work with a client on each stage sequentially. However, the rigid adherence to any model prevents therapists from being able to be supportive and available to the person with AIDS in a way that is more meaningful and responsive to the individual. In addition, the adherence to these models can engender in therapists increased feelings of failure and ineffectiveness if clients do not progress smoothly through the sequence of stages.

In order to minimize the painful awareness of their own mortality, and to reduce the anxiety associated with death, ther-apists sometimes unconsciously engage in such dangerous ac-tivities as minimization. They may minimize the seriousness of both medical symptoms and psychological distress, colluding with clients' own needs to avoid confronting these issues. They may not support, or actively discourage, individuals from deal-ing with painful topics, such as writing wills, saying goodbye to significant others, or making plans for a funeral. Even more dangerous is when a therapist's anxiety results in missing subtle communications from a client about suicidal ideations, despair, or withdrawal from their usual activities.

Overreaction may be another defense to the therapist's own anxiety when confronting issues of mortality. This may be man-ifested in a therapist's unnecessary alarm over a report of med-ical symptoms, or more critically, his or her inability to maintain availablility for clients when their medical status worsens. As a defense against feeling loss, a therapist may begin avoiding a client as he or she becomes more ill, rationalizing that "therapy" cannot be done during those periods.

In fact, when we begin to work with someone who is di-agnosed with AIDS, there is a danger of maintaining an even greater professional distance and detachment than we usually maintain. Though we may feel that this is professionally correct, it is possible that it is related to our fear of becoming attached to someone who may die. Much of our work is through a partial therapeutic identification. It may be more difficult to do this with people who have a life-threatening illness. We may stop the investment of ourselves because, instinctively, we do not want to lend ourselves to dying through identification.

Persons with AIDS have often had the experience of sig-nificant others withdrawing from them, rejecting them, or gen-erally being critical and negative, whether based on judgments about the illness or fear of the illness and contagion. The therapist who is afraid of loss or who believes it is professionally correct to stay distant and detached mirrors that same reaction in the therapeutic relationship.

Our own vulnerability in the face of losses, our feared losses, and existential anxiety about the nature of life and death may also mitigate against feeling hopeful in our work. This can lead, at the worst, to depression, phobic reactions, and burnout. On the other hand, we may continue trying to make a difference, and become compulsive and driven about our work—forgetting to balance life and living with death and dying. There is a tendency to feel that all else pales in front of issues of dying and death, so we continue to work even when we are overloaded and stressed.

As with more general issues of countertransference, any unusual response to a client may be a clue to our anxious or defensive involvement with that client. It is, perhaps, easier rationally to justify these defenses when working with someone who has AIDS. However, these unexamined defenses will inhibit or harm our therapeutic work with clients, whereas an understanding and exploration of these defenses may help us both to work more effectively and to understand what our clients may be experiencing.

Suggestions for Confronting Countertransference Issues and Preventing Burnout

Many of our suggestions have been implicit in the discussions of both factors influencing countertransference and the defenses therapists use. Most importantly, therapists must remain cognizant of the extra demands, stresses, and personal reactions they will encounter in working with persons with AIDS, especially those who are approaching death. Therapists must consistently and carefully monitor their motivations for working with people with AIDS, their stress levels, and emotional reactions to the work. Especially common may be denial or over-identification, both reactions leading to ineffective and possibly harmful therapeutic interventions.

It is important for us to make the distinction between being ineffective as therapists, and the realistic helplessness we all may feel in the face of death. We need to explore our own feelings about illness, dying and death, and our beliefs about the goals of therapeutic interventions in these situations. We may not be able to prevent someone from dying, but we may be able to help them feel less alone and misunderstood in that process.

Therapists who experience sadness and the pain of grief when a person with whom they are working dies need to validate these feelings and accept them as legitimate and appropriate. They must also find effective measures for coping with their own grief. It is important for people who work with AIDS to understand that experiencing grief and loss is not a failure of the therapeutic relationship, nor is it crossing over a professional boundary; rather it is a reflection of having had a genuine and real relationship with the person who is entering the final stages of his or her life. As such, it is not unusual for a therapist to want to attend a funeral or memorial service for someone who has died. This is not a reflection of overattachment or boundary-blurring, but rather may be a necessary step to validate a therapist's legitimate sense of loss. It is, however, not the only way to attain a sense of closure about people with whom therapists have worked who have died. What is important is that each therapist find a way to mourn his or her losses.

Therapists need to know when and with whom they can and cannot work without sacrificing their own quality of life. They may need to limit the number of clients with AIDS that they have in their case load at any one time. There may also be times that a therapist needs to accept that the work has become too difficult or painful, and not blame her- or himself or experience this as a professional failure. Rather, it may be a natural consequence of working in an area that constantly demands the experience of working through pain and loss.

Especially important to those working with persons with AIDS is the support and consultation of others doing similar work. Not only will this allow for the sharing of personal experiences, but may help facilitate identifying countertransference reactions of which the therapist is unaware.

Conclusion

We want to conclude this chapter with a personal statement by each of us about our work in this area. We hope that these statements will help illustrate some of the countertransference issues we have discussed above, and the ways we have attempted to work with or resolve these issues.

Scott Sherman: Reflecting upon my own experience and professional development in working with people who have AIDS, two experiences that clearly represent countertransference issues for me come to mind from the beginning of the work. The first was leading a therapy group, as part of a research project, with 12 men who had AIDS. Following the group they were asked to fill out some forms. Many of the men did not have pens; I happily loaned out mine for them to use. After everyone had finished and left the room, I was left with the pen several men with AIDS had used, and did not know what to do with it. I threw the pen out, fearful of even touching it. I realize now that I was overwhelmed by the experience of so many ill, dying men, who were not very different from myself, at a time when there was little hope of any treatment. In my anxiety about having to deal with issues and fears about death and dying, I could not touch them—either physically or emotionally—not even a pen they had touched. Thinking about my own fears, and my embarrassment at my own behavior, helped me to begin to examine what I would need to confront if I were going to be able to provide anything resembling therapy to these men. I am pleased that I found the support of colleagues at that time so that I am now able to hug someone with AIDS when it is needed, or to be with someone who is dying in the hospital, or simply hold someone's hand or stroke someone's arms to make sure the person knows and experiences my presence.

The second experience involved a man in his 30s, whom I had been seeing for 5 years in twice-weekly dynamic therapy. Around the same time as the group project, this man became ill with a rather aggressive form of lymphoma. We attempted to continue his treatment while he was in the hospital. He was convinced chemotherapy would wipe out his cancer, and the issue of AIDS was denied. "This is not AIDS, I have cancer" was his message. As he became more and more ill, and the cancer did not respond to chemotherapy, the doctors spoke with him directly about his condition, about AIDS, and about his poor prognosis. The client would then say to me things that clearly distorted what he had been told, and firmly denied his condition. I felt confused and wondered how to best work through this denial. For weeks, as his condition deteriorated, I walked a thin line between supporting his denial and confronting the issue of his certain death: it was excruciating to me. Finally, out of frustration stemming from all I had read about the stages of dying, I sought consultation. I felt I was clearly failing this man, after 5 years of work. I felt too close to him and too upset by his illness to help him come to terms with his death. In the consultation I was told, "Maybe he just can't say goodbye, and that is all right." I finally understood that my failure was in not allowing him to be where he was, and in not respecting and supporting what part, if any, of the "work" he could do. I began to feel free to be with him and allow him to decide how he would leave me, his family, and his friends. I believe that he truly appreciated my support. Until he went into a coma and died 2 days later, he believed he could beat his illness and that he did not have AIDS. This man's illness and death were powerful lessons for me, teaching me to respect and value the infinite number of ways people deal with their own death.

The impact of AIDS on me personally and professionally has been immense, and, at times, overwhelming. I have felt sadness as I watched vital, energetic men begin to wither away. I have felt pride seeing clients demonstrate courage, humor, and peace in the face of death and physical and emotional pain. I have feared for my health. This has been especially true when a client has had dementia or organic brain syndrome. I knew I would hate that type of illness the most, and would not want others to have to endure the pain of watching that process. I have feared for those I love, wondering if I could be there for them, or if they could be there for me. I have felt intense rage at the slowness of the government's reponse and at the total ignorance and bigotry of some people.

I have been challenged to find words of comfort for grieving lovers, mothers, family members, and friends, and have often doubted whether any words could bring comfort. I have received notes about the comfort I have been able to offer, and wondered what I had said, so that I could draw upon those words the next time. Usually I do not remember a word, reminding me that there is no formula.

Certainly, as simple as it sounds, working with people who have AIDS has helped me to think more carefully about my life, my choices, and my priorities. I value my time and guard it. I am more able to say no to professional opportunities, and set limits with myself, giving myself more personal time for being with the people I love. Mostly, I feel grateful that I have allowed people with AIDS to touch my life, as painful as that is at times. They have taught me much about grace, courage, and living.

Sheila Namir: I have been providing consultation and therapy to people with life-threatening illnesses for the past 7 years. In thinking about the impact of this work on my personal and professional life, I began to realize that I have gone through different periods in the process. At the beginning, I believe that I was counterphobic in my approach. Somehow, I magically believed that if I worked with people who were dying, I would be able to come to terms with fears about people I loved or my own potential for becoming ill or dying. There must also have been some unconscious belief that by contributing in this way, I, and those I cared about, would be protected from illness or dying.

As the work intensified, and I began to struggle with my own reactions to clients, I became overwhelmed by the grief I was feeling and unable to express. I remember a young woman with whom I felt particularly close and identified with because of similarities between us. She died while I was with her, and as I walked down 10 flights of stairs crying, only to emerge back into the hospital contained and professional, I realized that I had no way to integrate my human grief reactions into my ideas about my professional role. I remember, also, trying to talk to a supervisor about countertransference issues that were emerging in my work, and being handed an article to read. He clearly gave me the message that we were not to discuss these feelings, and that, as a professional, I could find all the help I needed in the literature.

There were periods during these first years when I felt despair and anger. Although at times I felt ineffective because of these feelings, I began to try to direct them into actions. I remember one client saying to me that if physicians couldn't cure him, they could at least treat him humanely. I began to work with physicians and nurses to help them deal with their own feelings that, I felt, must be preventing them from showing the compassion they experienced. I also became active in directing my anger at decision makers at various levels of government.

I watched myself use denial. When one of my clients was diagnosed with cancer I kept minimizing it, saying to myself that she would be fine, that it wasn't a serious cancer. I even watched myself blame her for having symptoms for several months and not telling me or going to see a physician. I blamed myself for not having dealt earlier and more effectively with her difficulty in expressing feelings, or for not noticing that she had lost some weight. I wanted to avoid her, believing that I could no longer work with her if she had cancer (we had been engaged in psychodynamic psychotherapy before her diagnosis). I was finally able to be fully available to her during her struggle with cancer after I began to recognize how shocking it was for me that someone in my private practice had developed a life-threatening illness, while I worked with people with AIDS in another setting (probably in the hope that I could isolate that part of life), and began to explore the countertransference issues, grapple with the professional role, and therapeutic decisions.

Then there was the bargaining that sometimes occurred. I remember that I placed a lot of my hope in one man who had AIDS. I believed he would live and that he would confirm for me my belief that this was not a universally fatal disease. I began to recognize that I was saying to myself, "I won't be able to bear it if he dies too." I recognized my countertransference when, after a particularly lively session with him, I began to imagine what I would say about him in eulogy, and realized the defensive aspect of this fantasy.

There are the funerals I went to, not knowing where to sit. I was not really friend or family. You can often tell who the therapist is at a funeral—she or he will be sitting alone in a pew in the back.

There were times that I couldn't go to the hospital, that I felt if one more person died I would not be able to continue this work, that the demands from clients, physicians, and friends were encroaching on the quality of my life.

I began to be intolerant of the daily demands, the ordinary problems in living, the neuroses of my clients. This was a phase where all else paled in the face of the trauma of a life-threatening illness. It also coincided with my intolerance of my own problems and pleasures—refusing to pay attention to my needs or feeling guilty if I enjoyed myself while my clients were suffering.

Eventually, by carefully exploring my reactions and the ways this work was affecting my life, I regained some perspective and balance in both my work and my personal life. I began to feel grateful and privileged to be allowed to do this work. Today I continue to learn from my clients about the meaning of life and of death and to confront my own beliefs more directly. I continue to be moved by the courage, integrity, and love I see in working with families, friends, and lovers of people with AIDS, as well as those struggling to live with AIDS. There are constant reminders to myself about what is really important and about the need to keep my priorities clear.

Eissler (1955, p. 245) asked, "Which is really harder—to die or to witness death?" I can't answer that, having experienced only the latter. But I can say that to witness is to participate, and to be forever changed by it.

References

Adler, G. (1972). Helplessness in the helpers. *British Journal of Medical Psychology*, *45*, 315–326.

Bascom, G.S. (1984). Physical, emotional, and cognitive care of dying patients. *Bulletin of the Menninger Clinic*, *48*, 351–356.

Burton, A. (1962). Death as a countertransference. *Psychoanalytic Review*, *49*, 3–20.

Clarke, P.J. (1981). Exploration of countertransference toward the dying. *American Journal of Orthopsychiatry*, *51*, 71–77.

Cohen, M.B. (1952). Countertransference and anxiety. *Psychiatry*, *15*, 231–243.

Eisendrath, S., & Dunkel, J. (1979). Psychological issues in intensive care unit staff. *Heart and Lung*, *8*, 751–758.

Eissler, K. (1955). *The psychiatrist and the dying patient*. New York: International Universities Press.

Freud, S. (1910). The future prospects of psychoanalytic therapy. *Standard Edition*, *11*, 141–151.

Gorkin, M. (1987). *The uses of countertransference*. Northvale, NJ: Jason Aronson.

Groves, J.E. (1978). Taking care of the hateful patient. *New England Journal of Medicine*, *298*, 883–887.

Heimann, P. (1950). On counter-transference. *International Journal of Psychoanalysis*, *31*, 81–84.

Kernberg, O.F. (1965). Notes on countertransference. *Journal of the American Psychoanalytic Association*, *13*, 38–54.

Kübler-Ross, E. (1969). *On death and dying*. New York: Macmillan.

Lindemann, E. (1944). Symptomatology and management of acute grief. *American Journal of Psychiatry*, *101*, 141–148.

Little, M. (1951). Counter-transference and the patient's response to it. *International Journal of Psychoanalysis*, *33*, 32–40.

Maltsberger, J.T., & Buie, D.H. (1974). Countertransference hate in the treatment of suicidal patients. *Archives of General Psychiatry*, *30*, 625–633.

Mandel, J.S. (1986). Psychosocial challenges of AIDS and ARC: Clinical research observations. In L. McKusick (Ed.), *What to do about AIDS* (pp. 75–86). Berkeley: University of California Press.

280 No Longer Immune

Namir, S., & Wellisch, D.W. (1985). The hated adolescent: Reactions of family and hospital staff to an aplastic anemia patient. *Family Systems Medicine, 3*, 313–325.

Pruyser, P.W. (1984). Existential impact of professional exposure to life-threatening or terminal illness. *Bulletin of the Menninger Clinic, 48*, 357–367.

Racker, H. (1957). The meanings and uses of countertransference. *Psychoanalytic Quarterly, 26*, 303–357.

Rando, T.A. (1984). *Grief, dying and death: Clinical interventions for caregivers.* Champaigne, IL: Research Press Co.

Renneker, R.E. (1957). Countertransference reactions to cancer. *Psychosomatic Medicine, 14*, 409–414.

Ryan, W. (1971). *Blaming the victim.* New York: Random House.

Sourkes, B.M. (1982). *The deepening shade: Psychological aspects of life-threatening illness.* Pittsburgh: University of Pittsburgh Press.

Weigert, E. (1954). Countertransference and self-analysis of the psychoanalyst. *International Journal of Psychoanalysis, 35*, 242–246.

Weisman, A.D. (1981). Understanding the cancer patient: The syndrome of caregivers' plight. *Psychiatry, 44*, 161–168.

LIST OF CONTRIBUTORS

Alicia Boccellari, PhD, is the director of Neuropsychology Service at San Francisco General Hospital and is assistant clinical professor of psychology at University of California San Francisco, Department of Psychiatry, School of Medicine. Dr. Boccellari has been actively involved in working with individuals with AIDS dementia complex and their caregivers. She has been involved in conducting research at San Francisco General Hospital on the natural history and course of AIDS dementia complex.

David Cramer, PhD, has been involved as an educator, practitioner, and volunteer in helping people cope with AIDS since 1984. As a psychologist, he has counseled individuals, couples, and families affected by the HIV. In addition, he has facilitated a PWA group and presented numerous programs on AIDS in the work place. Volunteer efforts have included community lectures, becoming a "buddy" to a PWA, and presently serving as a buddy trainer. Dr. Cramer is the program director for Group Services at the Counseling and Mental Health Center of The University of Texas at Austin. He also maintains a private practice.

John H. Curtis, PhD, is a professor of sociology and anthropology at Valdosta State College, where he coordinates an AIDS research project. He is a founding member of the National Coalition on AIDS and Families, a member of the Groves Conference Task Force on AIDS, and the National Conference on Family Relations (NCFR) Task Force on AIDS. He has recently chaired the NCFR subgroup on AIDS and Religion. Dr. Curtis is active as a member of the District Eight Task Force on AIDS (Georgia Department of Public Health) and director of therapy for Wellness Associates Incorporated, a nonprofit association providing confidential services to persons with AIDS in southern Georgia.

Carole Donovan, RN, MA, is a home care nurse with the Supportive Care Program at St. Vincent's Hospital and Medical Center in New York City. She began her association with the program as a volunteer in 1980. Ms. Donovan was graduated from the University of Connecticut School of Nursing and received her master's degree from Teacher's College, Columbia University. Her long-standing interest in hospice began in 1967 when she heard Cicely Saunders describe her work at St. Christopher's Hospice, England. Several years later, Ms. Donovan participated in a work-study program there. She has also served as a board member at the Connecticut Hospice, Inc., Branford.

Maria Ekstrand, PhD, received her PhD in clinical psychology from Auburn University, Alabama, in 1986. Following completion of a clinical internship at the University of Mississippi Medical Center, Jackson, MS, Dr. Ekstrand held a postdoctoral research position in health psychology at the University of California, San Francisco (UCSF). She currently works as assistant research psychologist in the Center for AIDS Prevention Studies and the Department of Epidemiology at UCSF where she is conducting secondary analyses of data on psychosocial aspects of AIDS and AIDS prevention. Her work includes a fellowship grant from the American Foundation for AIDS Research (AmFar) and a NICHHD grant to study biopsychosocial predictors of high-risk sexual behavior among adolescents in detention at the San Francisco Youth Guidance Center.

Nancy J. Garfield, PhD, received her PhD in counseling psychology from the University of Missouri-Columbia, and is a licensed psychologist and the director of training, Psychology Service at Colmery-O'Neil Veterans Administration Medical Center, Topeka, Kansas. At the hospital she provides HIV test counseling, AIDS education for patients and staff, and is on AIDS-related committees. She was the vice-chair of the board of directors of the Topeka AIDS Project and their education director. She has chaired several regional AIDS conferences and made numerous presentations about AIDS on topics ranging from ethical issues for clergy and other human development specialists to basic AIDS transmission information.

Richard Green, MD, JD, is professor in residence in the School of Medicine and in the School of Law at the University of California, Los Angeles (UCLA). Dr. Green received his medical degree from the Johns Hopkins University and his law degree from Yale. He has been editor-in-chief of the *Archives of Sexual Behavior* since its inception in 1971 and was the founding president of the International Academy of Sex Research. His books include the co-edited *Transsexualism and Sex Reassignment*, the edited *Human Sexuality: A Health Practitioner's Text* (two editions), the co-authored *Impotence*, and two authored books, *Sexual Identity Conflict in Children and Adults* and *The "Sissy Boy Syndrome" and the Development of Homosexuality*.

Joseph R. Guydish, PhD, completed doctoral training in clinical psychology at Washington State University in 1987. While an intern at Langley Porter Psychiatric Institute, and later as a postdoctoral fellow in the Department of Psychiatry at the University of California, San Francisco (UCSF), Dr. Guydish specialized in the area of behavioral medicine. During this time he worked extensively with HIV-affected patients in clinical practice, and developed research interests in HIV-related risk behavior change. Dr. Guydish is currently a visiting postgraduate scholar in the Center for AIDS Prevention Studies, UCSF, researching risk behavior in heterosexual and intravenous drug-using populations.

The Reverend James A. Hammond is an Episcopal priest with 17 years of experience in parochial and scholastic settings. He holds a bachelor of arts degree from the University of Maryland, College Park, and a master of divinity degree from Seabury-Western Theological Seminary, Evanston, Illinois. He has been active in AIDS education and prevention for most of the 1980s, giving particular emphasis to people and programs at the parish level. The Rev. Hammond served as a member of the board of directors of the Topeka AIDS Project, Topeka, Kansas.

Sally Jue, LCSW, is a licensed clinical social worker and the mental health director at AIDS Project Los Angeles. In addition to her duties there, she has lectured at several professional conferences on the mental health aspect of AIDS, participated on the California State AIDS Leadership Team's Mental Health Committee, and the Surgeon General's national AIDS mailing and public service announcements. She has also published articles on cross-cultural counseling and AIDS and on identifying and meeting the needs of the minority client with AIDS.

Craig D. Kain, holds a Ph.D. in counseling psychology at the University of Southern California. Mr. Kain serves as an ad hoc reviewer for the American Association for Counseling and Development's *Journal of Counseling and Development*. Mr. Kain maintains a private counseling practice where he works with many HIV-infected men. He has also presented numerous trainings and papers for counselors on AIDS. Mr. Kain is an adjunct faculty member of Antioch University, Los Angeles.

Grant Knapp-Duncan is currently a consultant to Bay Area Addiction Research and Treatment, Inc, in San Francisco while pursuing a master's degree in social work. Since receiving his BSW from the University of Missouri, he has worked with substance users, developmentally disabled adults, geriatric patients in long-term care facilities, and with people with AIDS. Mr. Knapp-Duncan is a member of the National Association of Social Workers.

Ted Knapp-Duncan has been research director at Youth Environment Study, Inc., and Mid-City Consortium to Combat AIDS in San Francisco since 1988. Formerly he served as counselor supervisor at the Alternate Test Site in San Francisco's Castro District under the auspices of the Psychiatry Department, University of California, and as professor of health administration at the University of Kansas Medical Center. His clinical research interests have included people with HIV disease, type II diabetes, chronic pain, and cancer. Dr. Knapp-Duncan received his BA from the University of California at Berkeley and his PhD in psychology from the University of Tennessee at Knoxville. He is a member of the American Public Health Association.

Sister Patrice Murphy, RN, MS, is the director of the Supportive Care Program at St. Vincent's Hospital and Medical Center, New York City, and has been a member of the Sisters of Charity since 1950. She graduated from St. Vincent's School of Nursing and received her master's degree from Hunter College of the City of New York. Sr. Murphy has been active in nursing service and education since 1956 and is a member of the National Association of Catholic Chaplains. Sr. Murphy has been actively involved in the AIDS crisis since 1983 and is a board member of the AIDS Resource Center and Pax Christi Hospice.

Sheila Namir, PhD, is associate professor at the California School of Professional Psychology (CSPP) and assistant clinical professor at University of California, Los Angeles (UCLA) Department of Psychiatry and Biobehavioral Sciences. She was a co-investigator and director of the UCLA Psychosocial AIDS Study from 1983–1986, and currently is an investigator for the Women and AIDS Risk Network project at CSPP, a prevention and education program funded by the National Institute on Drug Abuse. Dr. Namir has published many clinical and research articles on the psychosocial aspects of AIDS, and has presented workshops, trainings, and papers on AIDS. She is also a clinical psychologist practicing psychology in Los Angeles.

Margaret Nichols, PhD, received her PhD in clinical psychology from Columbia University Teacher's College in 1981. She is currently the executive director of the Institute for Personal Growth, Inc., a counseling and therapy center geared primarily, though not exclusively, to the gay, lesbian, and bisexual community. Dr. Nichols is the founding executive director of the Hyacinth Foundation AIDS Project, the first and largest not-for-profit organization in New Jersey to deliver psychosocial services to people with AIDS, their partners, relatives, and friends.

The Reverend Albert J. Ogle is a priest of the Anglican Church of Ireland. He was awarded his divinity degree with honors by University College of North Wales. He did further theological study at Trinity College, Dublin, the Universtiy of London Institute of Education, and the University of Ireland at Maynooth. The Reverend Ogle has served parishes in Belfast and Dublin, directed an inner city project in London, and was licensed to officiate in the Diocese of Los Angeles in 1982. He has held staff positions at the Gay and Lesbian Community Services Center in Hollywood, California and was founder of the Triangle Project for high-risk youth. The Reverend Ogle was director of planning and development at AIDS Project Los Angeles and initiated and developed the AIDS Interfaith Council of Southern California. He is co-author of the "Myers Plan," a statewide needs assessment and plan for AIDS treatment services in California for 1987–1991, published by the Health Policy and Research Foundation of California. He has been a consultant with the Episcopal Commission on AIDS Ministry for the Diocese of Los Angeles, and, since 1987, has been executive director of the All Saints AIDS Service Center in Pasadena, California.

Scott Sherman, PhD, is a clinical psychologist in private practice. Since 1982, when he began to serve as a consultant to the then three-person staff of AIDS Project Los Angeles, he has been providing direct clinical services to persons with AIDS, ARC, and their significant others. In addition, Dr. Sherman has provided training in the psychosocial aspects of AIDS throughout the state of California to mental health professionals. Most recently, Dr. Sherman has been providing workshops for professionals dealing with issues of transference and countertransference as they affect working with AIDS, grief, and loss.

Barbara R. Slater, PhD, is professor of psychology and coordinator of school psychology at Towson State University, Towson, Maryland. She maintains a private practice, specializing in working with children and women. Dr. Slater is a diplomate in school psychology of the American Board of Professional Psychology, a fellow of the American Psychological Association, and past president of the Division of School Psychology of the American Psychological Association. She is a member of the Presidential Task Force on AIDS on the campus at Towson State University and a member of the Preliminary Consortium on Services to Sexual Minority Youth of the state of Maryland Department of Health and Mental Hygiene.

Michael D. Shore, PhD, is director of the Neuropsychology Service at the Transitions Head Injury Program in Berkeley, California. He is also adjunct faculty at the California School of Professional Psychology, Berkeley. Dr. Shore is a clinical and research consultant to the Neropsychology Service at San Francisco General Hospital and is active in research investigating the impact of AIDS on the central nervous system.

RESOURCES FOR COUNSELORS

Following is a list of resources for counselors. The list is divided into three sections covering community-based AIDS service organizations, U.S. governmental agencies, and national private sector agencies. This list was compiled using "AIDS Lifeline," the National AIDS Network Directory of AIDS Education and Service Organizations.

The National AIDS Network supports over 550 organizations that provide community-based AIDS education and services. The agency, headquartered in Washington, DC, was formed in 1985 as a private, not-for-profit organization by five of the nation's pioneering community-based AIDS service agencies, and acts as a conduit for service providers to share hands-on experience and receive technical expertise. The National AIDS Network also acts as a clearinghouse for information and programs.

COMMUNITY-BASED AIDS SERVICE ORGANIZATIONS

Alabama
AIDS Task Force of Alabama
P.O. Box 55703
Birmingham, AL 35255
Phone: 205-322-0757
Local Hotline: 205-930-3741
Toll-Free Hotline: 800-445-3741

Alaska
Alaska AIDS Project
P.O. Box 200070
Anchorage, AK 99520
Phone: 907-276-4880
Local Hotline: 907-276-4880
Toll-Free Hotline: 800-478-AIDS

Arizona
Arizona AIDS Project
736 East Flynn Lane
Phoenix, AZ 85014
Phone: 602-277-1929
Local Hotline: 602-277-1929

Tucson AIDS Project
151 South Tucson Boulevard, Suite 252
Tucson, AZ 85745
Phone: 602-322-6226
Local Hotline: 602-326-AIDS

Arkansas
Arkansas AIDS Foundation
P.O. Box 5007
Little Rock, AR 72225
Phone: 501-224-4020
Local Hotline: 501-374-5503

California
AIDS Project Los Angeles
3670 Wilshire Blvd., Suite 300
Los Angeles, CA 90010
Phone: 213-380-2000
Local Hotline: 213-876-AIDS
Toll-Free Hotline: 800-922-AIDS

San Diego AIDS Project
P.O. Box 89049
San Diego, CA 92138
Phone: 619-543-0300

AIDS Health Project
Box 0884
San Francisco, CA 94143-0884
Phone: 415-476-6430

San Francisco AIDS Foundation
Box 6182
San Francisco, CA 94101-6128
Phone: 415-864-4376
Toll-Free Hotline: 800-FOR-AIDS
Hearing Impaired Information: 415-
864-6606 (TTY)

Shanti Foundation
9060 Santa Monica Blvd., Suite 301
West Hollywood, CA 90069
Phone: 213-272-7591

Shanti Foundation
525 Howard Street
San Francisco, CA 94105
Phone: 415-777-2273

Colorado
Boulder County AIDS Project
P.O. Box 4375
Boulder, CO 80306
Phone: 303-444-6121

Colorado AIDS Project
P.O. Box 18529
Denver, CO 80218
Phone: 303-837-0166

Connecticut
AIDS Project Hartford
30 Arbor Street
Hartford, CT 06106
Phone: 203-523-7699
Local Hotline: 203-247-AIDS
                203-951-SIDA (Spanish)

AIDS Project New Haven
P.O. Box 636
New Haven, CT 06503
Phone: 203-624-2437

Delaware
Delaware Lesbian and Gay Health
  Advocates
214 North Market
Wilmington, DE 19802
Phone: 302-652-6776
Local Hotline: 302-655-5280
Toll-Free Hotline: 800-422-0429

District of Columbia
Whitman-Walker Clinic/AIDS Program
1407 S Street, N.W., 4th floor
Washington, DC 20009
Phone: 202-332-5295
Local Hotline: 202-322-2437
Hearing Impaired Information: 202-
  332-5295 (TDD)

Florida
Daytona AIDS Resources and Education
  (DARE)
P.O. Box 9306
Daytona Beach, FL 32020
Phone: 904-257-4208
Local Hotline: 904-257-4208

AIDS Center One
370 East Prospect Road
Fort Lauderdale, FL 33334
Phone: 305-561-0316
Local Hotline: 305-561-0316
Toll-Free Hotline: 800-325-5371

AID Jacksonville
1919 Beachway Road, Suite 5D
Jacksonville, FL 32207
Phone: 904-399-4589

Health Crisis Network
P.O. Box 42-1280
Miami, FL 33242-1280
Phone: 305-326-8833
305-324-5248 (Spanish)
Local Hotline: 305-634-4436
Toll-Free Hotline: 800-443-5046

Georgia
AIDS Athens, Inc.
1382 Prince Avenue, Suite 96
Athens, GA 30606
Phone: 404-542-2437

AIDS Atlanta
1132 West Peachtree, NW
Atlanta, GA 30309-3624
Phone: 404-872-0600
Local Hotline: 404-876-9944
Toll-Free Hotline: 800-551-2728
Hearing Impaired Information: 404-876-9950 (TTY)

Georgia AIDS Action Committee
P.O. Box 7482
Atlanta, GA 30357

Central City AIDS Network
P.O. Box 6452
Macon, GA 31208
Phone: 912-742-2437

Hawaii
Life Foundation
P.O. Box 89980
Honolulu, HI 96830-8980
Phone: 808-924-2437

Idaho
Idaho AIDS Foundation
P.O. Box 421
Boise, ID 83701-0421
Phone: 208-345-2277
Local Hotline: 208-345-2277

Illinois
Gay Community AIDS Project
P.O. Box 713
Champaign, IL 61820
Phone: 217-337-2928
Local Hotline: 217-351-2437

AIDS Foundation of Chicago
2035 East Superior, Passavant 5 West
Chicago, IL 60611
Phone: 312-908-9191
Local Hotline: 312-908-9191

AIDS Foundation of Chicago
2035 North Lincoln Ave., Suite 619
Chicago, IL 60614
Phone: 312-525-9466

Indiana
AIDS Task Force
P.O. Box 13527
Fort Wayne, IN 46869
Phone: 219-484-2711

Marion County AIDS Coalition
1350 North Pennsylvania Street, Damien
Center
Indianapolis, IN 46220
Phone: 317-634-1441
Local Hotline: 317-257-HOPE

Iowa
Rapids AIDS Project
P.O. Box 2861
Cedar Rapids, IA 52406
Phone: 319-395-7530

AIDS Education Committee/Gay
Coalition of Des Moines
P.O. Box 851
Des Moines, IA 50304

Central Iowa AIDS Project
2116 Grand Avenue
Des Moines, IA 50132
Phone: 515-274-6700
Toll-Free Hotline: 800-445-AIDS

IOWA Center for AIDS/ARC Resources
and Education
P.O. Box 2989
Iowa City, IA 52244
Phone: 319-338-5508

Kansas
Kansas AIDS Network
P.O. Box 2727
Topeka, KS 66601
Phone: 913-367-7499
Local Hotline: 913-357-7499
Toll-Free Hotline: 800-255-1382

Topeka AIDS Project
P.O. Box 118
Topeka, KS 66601
Phone: 913-232-3100
Local Hotline: 913-232-3100

Kentucky
AIDS Crisis Taskforce
P.O. Box 11442
Lexington, KY 40575
Phone: 606-281-5151

AIDS Program—Louisville Urban
  League
2600 West Broadway, Lyles Mall—3rd
  Floor
Louisville, KY 40211
Phone: 502-776-4622

Louisiana
No/AIDS Task Force
P.O. Box 2616
New Orleans, LA 70176-2616
Phone: 504-891-3732
Local Hotline: 504-522-2437
Toll-Free Hotline: 800-992-4379

New Orleans AIDS Project
1231 Prytania Street
New Orleans, LA 70130
Phone: 504-523-3755

Maine
AIDS Project
48 Deering Street
Portland, ME 04101
Phone: 207-774-6877
Local Hotline: 207-775-1267
Toll-Free Hotline: 800-851-AIDS

Maryland
AIDS Response Network
1315 North Charles Street
Baltimore, MD 21201
Phone: 301-837-AIDS
Local Hotline: 301-837-AIDS

Health Education Resource
  Organization (HERO)
101 West Read Street, Suite 812
Baltimore, MD 21201
Phone: 301-685-1180
Local Hotline: 301-685-1180
Toll-Free Hotline: 800-638-6252
Hearing Impaired Information: 800-
  553-3140 (TTY)

Massachusetts
AIDS Action
661 Boylston Street, Suite 4
Boston, MA 02116
Phone: 617-437-6200
Local Hotline: 617-536-7733
Toll-Free Hotline: 800-235-2331
Hearing Impaired Information: 617-
  536-7733 (TTY)

Michigan
AIDS Phone Network/ Wayne County
  Medical Society
1010 Antietam
Detroit, MI 48207
Phone: 313-567-1640

Grand Rapids AIDS Task Force
P.O. Box 6603
Grand Rapids, MI 49516
Phone: 616-956-9009
Local Hotline: 616-956-9009

Minnesota
Minnesota AIDS Project
2025 Nicollet Avenue, South, Suite 200
Minneapolis, MN 55404
Phone: 612-870-7773
Local Hotline: 612-870-0700
Toll-Free Hotline: 800-248-AIDS

Mississippi
Mississippi Gay Alliance
P.O. Box 8324
Jackson, MS 39204
Phone: 601-353-7611

Missouri
Mid Missouri AIDS Project
811 East Cherry, Room 321, P.O. Box
  1371
Columbia, MO 65202
Phone: 314-875-2437

Metropolitan St. Louis AIDS Program
634 North Grand Boulevard
St. Louis, MO 63103
Phone: 314-658-1159

St. Louis Effort For AIDS
4050 Lindell Blvd.
St. Louis, MO 63108
Phone: 314-531-2847
Local Hotline: 314-531-7400

Montana
Billings AIDS Support Network
P.O. Box 1748
Billings, MT 59103
Phone: 406-252-1212
Local Hotline: 406-252-1212
Toll-Free Hotline: 800-537-6187

Nebraska
Nebraska AIDS Project
3624 Leavenworth
Omaha, NE 68105
Phone: 402-342-4233
Toll-Free Hotline: 800-782-2437

Nevada
AIDS For AIDS of Nevada
2116 Paradise Road, Suites C & D
Las Vegas, NV 89104
Phone: 702-369-6162

Nevada AIDS Foundation
P.O. Box 478
Reno, NV 89504
Phone: 702-329-2437

New Hampshire
New Hampshire AIDS Foundation
P.O. Box 59
Manchester, NH 03105
Phone: 603-595-0218

New Jersey
South Jersey Against AIDS
1616 Pacific Avenue
Atlantic City, NJ 08401
Phone: 609-348-2437

Hyacinth Foundation AIDS Project
211 Livingston Avenue
New Brunswick, NJ 08901
Phone: 201-246-0925
Toll-Free Hotline: 800-433-0254

New Mexico
New Mexico AIDS Services
124 Quincy, NE
Albuquerque, NM 87108
Phone: 505-266-0911

New York
AIDS Council of Northeastern New
  York
307 Hamilton Street
Albany, NY 12210
Phone: 518-434-4686
Local Hotline: 518-445-AIDS

Western New York AIDS Program
220 Delaware Avenue, Suite 512
Buffalo, NY 14202
Phone: 716-847-AIDS

Gay Men's Health Crisis, Inc.
129 West 20th Street
New York, NY 10011
Phone: 212-807-6655
Local Hotline: 212-807-6655

Stop AIDS Project of New York
1123 Broadway, Suite 1205
New York, NY 10001
Phone: 212-645-0519

AIDS Task Force of Central New York
P.O. Box 1911
Syracuse, NY 13201
Phone: 315-475-2430
Local Hotline: 315-875-AIDS

North Carolina
Western North Carolina (WNC) AIDS
  Project
P.O. Box 2411
Asheville, NC 28802-2411
Phone: 704-252-7489
Local Hotline: 704-252-7489

AIDS Task Force of Winston-Salem
P.O. Box 2982
Winston-Salem, NC 27102
Phone: 919-723-5031
Local Hotline: 919-723-5031

North Dakota
The Coalition
1112 West Capital Avenue #127
Bismarck, ND 58501
Phone: 701-258-7166

Ohio
Multi-County AIDS Network
P.O. Box 1523
Akron, OH 44309
Phone: 216-762-8144

AIDS Volunteer of Cincinnati
P.O. Box 19009
Cincinnati, OH 45219
Phone: 513-421-2437

Western Reserve AIDS Foundation
1001 Huron Road, 10th Floor
Cleveland, OH 44115
Phone: 216-621-9723

Columbus AIDS Task Force
P.O. Box 8393
Columbus, OH 43201
Phone: 614-488-2437
Local Hotline: 614-224-0411

Area AIDS Task Force, Inc.
P.O. Box 342
Toledo, OH 43693-0342
Phone: 419-243-9351

Oklahoma
Oasis Community Center/AIDS Support
    Program
2135 NW 39th Street
Oklahoma City, OK 73112
Phone: 405-525-AIDS
Local Hotline: 405-525-AIDS

Tulsa AIDS Task Force
1412 East 38th Street, P.O. Box 4330
Tulsa, OK 74105
Phone: 918-584-4093

Oregon
Willamette AIDS Council
329 West 13th Avenue, Suite D
Eugene, OR 97401
Phone: 503-345-7089
Local Hotline: 503-345-7089

Cascade AIDS Project
408 WS 2nd, Suite 412
Portland, OR 97204
Phone: 503-223-5907
Local Hotline: 503-223-AIDS
Toll-Free Hotline: 800-777-AIDS

Oregon AIDS Task Force
P.O. Box 40104
Portland, OR 97240
Phone: 503-254-8812

Pennsylvania
AIDS Service Center
P.O. Box 1656
Allentown, PA 18105
Phone: 215-435-4616

South Central AIDS Assistance Network
    (SCAAN)
P.O. Box 11573
Harrisburg, PA 17108
Phone: 717-236-4772

Philadelphia AIDS Task Force
P.O. Box 53429
Philadelphia, PA 19107

Philadelphia Community Health
    Alternatives
P.O. Box 53429
Philadelphia, PA 19105
Phone: 215-732-2437
Local Hotline: 215-732-AIDS

Pittsburgh AIDS Task Force
141 South Highland Avenue, Suite 304
Pittsburgh, PA 15206
Phone: 412-363-6500
Local Hotline: 412-363-2437

Puerto Rico
Fundacion SIDA De Puerto Rico
GPO Box 4842
San Juan, PR 00926-4842
Phone: 809-751-4200

Rhode Island
Rhode Island Project AIDS
Roger Williams Bldg.
22 Hayes Street
Providence, RI 02908
Phone: 401-277-6545
Local Hotline: 401-277-6502

South Carolina
Carolina AIDS Research and Education
    (CARE)
U.S.C. School of Public Health
Columbia, SC 29208
Phone: 803-777-2273

South Dakota
Sioux Empire Gay and Lesbian Coalition
P.O. Box 220
Sioux Falls, SD 57101
Phone: 605-332-4599

Tennessee
Tri-Cities AIDS Project
P.O. Box 231
Johnson City, TN 37605

AIDS Response Knoxville
P.O. Box 3932
Knoxville, TN 37927
Phone: 615-523-2437
Local Hotline: 615-523-AIDS

Memphis AIDS Coalition
1400 Central Avenue
Memphis, TN 38104
Phone: 901-726-1690

Vanderbilt AIDS Project
CCC 5319, Medical Center North
Vanderbilt University
Nashville, TN 37232
Phone: 615-322-2252

Texas
AIDS Services of Austin
P.O. Box 4874
Austin, TX 78765
Phone: 512-474-2273
Local Hotline: 512-472-2437

AIDS Arms Network
P.O. Box 190945
Dallas, TX 75219
Phone: 214-521-5191

AIDS Foundation Houston, Inc.
3927 Essex Lane
Houston, TX 77027
Phone: 713-623-6796
Local Hotline: 713-524-AIDS

San Antonio AIDS Foundation
P.O. Box 120113
San Antonio, TX 78212
Phone: 512-821-6218

Utah
AIDS Project Utah
P.O. Box 8485
Salt Lake City, UT 84108
Phone: 801-583-1300

Vermont
Vermont Cares
P.O. Box 5248
Burlington, VT 05402
Phone: 802-863-2437

Virginia
Alexandria AIDS Task Force
29 West Myrtle Street
Alexandria, VA 22301

AIDS Support Group
P.O. Box 2322
Charlottesville, VA 22902
Phone: 804-979-7714

Richmond AIDS Information Network
1721 Hanover Avenue
Richmond, VA 23219
Phone: 804-355-4428
Local Hotline: 804-358-2437

Washington
AIDS Prevention Project
1116 Summit Avenue, Suite 200
Seattle, WA 98101
Phone: 206-296-4999
Local Hotline: 206-296-4999

Seattle AIDS Action Committee
700 A East Pike
Seattle, WA 98122
Phone: 206-323-1229

Seattle AIDS Support Group
102 15th Avenue East
Seattle, WA 98112
Phone: 206-322-2437

Spokane AIDS Network (SPAN)
West 1801 Broadway, Suite 203
Spokane, WA 99201
Phone: 509-326-2467

West Virginia
AIDS Support Group/Help Center
c/o St. John's 1105 Quarrier Street
Charleston, WV 25301
Phone: 808-345-HOPE

Mountain State AIDS Network
P.O. Box 1401
Morgantown, WV 26501
Local Hotline: 304-599-6726

AIDS Task Force of the Upper Ohio
  Valley
99 1/2 12th Street, Suite 1
Wheeling, WV 26003

Wisconsin
Madison AIDS Support Network
P.O. Box 731
Madison, WI 53701-0731
Phone: 608-255-1711

Milwaukee AIDS Project
P.O. Box 92505
Milwaukee, WI 53202
Phone: 414-273-2437

Wyoming
Wyoming AIDS Project
P.O. Box 9353
Casper, WY 82602
Phone: 307-237-7833
Local Hotline: 307-237-7833

U.S. GOVERNMENT AGENCIES

Alcohol Drug Abuse and Mental Health Administration
National Institutes of Health
Building 10, Room 4N-224
9000 Rockville Pike
Bethesda, MD 20892
Phone: 301-496-5608
Peter Bridges, MD
Deputy AIDS Coordinator

Centers for Disease Control
1600 Clifton Road
Atlanta, GA 30333
Phone: 404-329-1374
Walter Dowdle
Deputy Director for AIDS

Centers for Disease Control
AIDS Education and Prevention
1600 Clifton Road
Atlanda, GA 30333
Phone: 404-639-2384
Fred Kroger
Acting Director

Centers for Disease Control
AIDS Epidemiology Branch
1600 Clifton Road
Atlanta, GA 30333
Phone: 404-329-3162
Harold Jaffe, MD
Chief

Centers for Disease Control
AIDS Program
1600 Clifton Road
Atlanta, GA 30333
Phone: 404-329-2405
James Curran
Director

Food and Drug Administration
Parklawn Building Room 1472
5600 Fishers Lane
Rockville, MD 20857
Phone: 301-443-1544
Frank Young
Commissioner

Health and Human Services, Department of
Hubert H. Humphrey Building
200 Independence Avenue, SW, Room
  716G
Washington, DC 20201
Phone: 202-245-7684
Robert Windom, MD
Assistant Secretary for Health

National AIDS Information Clearinghouse
Centers for Disease Control
P.O. Box 6003
Rockville, MD 20850
Phone: 301-251-5000
Ruthanne Blates
Project Director

NATIONAL PRIVATE-SECTOR ORGANIZATIONS

AIDS Action Council (AAC)
2033 M Street, 8th Floor
Washington, DC 20036
Phone: 202-547-3101

American Foundation for AIDS Research (AmFar)
40 West 57th Street, Suite 406
New York, NY 10019
Phone: 212-333-3118

Intergovernmental Health Policy Project (GWU)
2100 Pennsylvania Avenue, NW
Washington, DC 20037
Phone: 202-872-1445

National AIDS Network (NAN)
2033 M Street, Suite 800
Washington, DC 20036
Phone: 202-293-2437

National Association of People With AIDS (NAPWA)
2025 I Street, NW, Suite 415
Washington, DC 20006
Phone: 202-429-2856

National Leadership Coalition on AIDS (NaLCOA)
1150 17th Street, NW, Suite 202
Washington, DC 20036
Phone: 202-429-0930

National Lesbian and Gay Health Foundation (NLGHF)
P.O. Box 65472
Washington, DC 20036
Phone: 202-797-3708

National Minority AIDS Council (NMAC)
714 G Street, SE
Washington, DC 20003
Phone: 202-544-1076